COMPASSIONATE CARE: A PRACTICAL HANDBOOK FOR DEMENTIA CAREGIVING

NAVIGATING THE FINANCIAL. LEGAL, AND TECHNOLOGICAL ASPECTS OF CARE

L.E. SUMMERS

DEDICATION

To my dearest mother,

*This book is a tribute to your unwavering strength and the love that
flowed through you. As I delve through the depths of dementia, I am
reminded of our journey together—the highs and lows, the moments of
confusion and clarity, and the unbreakable bond we shared.*

*You faced the relentless grip of dementia with courage and grace,
teaching me the true meaning of resilience. Through your unwavering
spirit, you taught me the power of embracing each day, no matter how
challenging it became. Your unwavering love and determination
inspired me to embark on this journey of understanding, to shed light
on the complexities of dementia.*

*In this book, I strive to honor your memory and the countless others
who have faced this formidable foe. I hope that by sharing our story, I
can offer solace, guidance, and a glimmer of hope to those who are
navigating this path.*

*Mom, your legacy lives on in every word of this book. You may have
been taken from us by dementia's grip, but your spirit endures in my*

heart. Through this book, I hope to raise awareness to help bring a world where no one faces dementia alone.

This dedication is a testament to the extraordinary woman you were—a beacon of love, strength, and resilience. Thank you for the indelible mark you left on my life, and may your light continue to shine brightly, illuminating the path for others who face the challenges of dementia.

I will always love you, Mom.

I also would like to take a moment to thank those important people in my life who helped me to create this tribute. A special thank you to my children Tyler and Miles, and to their mother Iseabail Lane. I don't think I could have done this without their help.

INTRODUCTION

Please keep in mind that this book is based on my personal experience and research as I discuss the best options related to healthcare insurance, financial decisions, or legal matters. It is my goal to offer helpful and accurate information, but I am not a medical professional or insurance specialist. No advice offered is a substitute for the expert guidance of a professional. My primary message throughout this book is to recommend that you consult with a healthcare professional, insurance specialist, or financial advisor for their specialized knowledge. The well-being of your loved one relies on us to do our best. Also, keep in mind that regulations and insurance plans vary by location and may also change over time.

At first, it can be hard to note the signs of dementia in your loved one. It starts with them repeatedly forgetting little things, like a keychain or a wallet. You will notice overdue bills coming in the mail and that they are having trouble remembering the names of things. These small lapses may be the first signs that things will be changing from now on.

Even with all these signs, it's hard to be prepared to hear the dementia diagnosis from a doctor. In a nutshell, it means that the mind of the person you love is starting to fade and, with time, won't be able to recognize their loved ones and will lose a sense of who they are. All sorts of scenarios may come to mind in this situation, but this is the time to be calm and practical and start making plans.

The caregiver is often a family member who looks after the patient with dementia in their daily lives. They are also responsible for keeping the rest of the family informed about the progress of the disease. Watching the cognitive decline of your loved one while grappling with grief, guilt, and a range of other complex emotions can lead you toward making wrong decisions. Taking care of a patient with dementia is an act of love, but it also requires planning and reasoning. Each financial decision a caregiver makes can have an impact on the dignity and peace of mind of everyone involved.

Not everyone decides to become a caregiver. As the first signs of dementia appear, you may find yourself in the middle of a storm that you aren't prepared to face. Finding focus and peace of mind isn't always easy, and it becomes harder when you don't know how to spend your money, or theirs, and deal with all the issues that lie ahead.

In this book, those starting their caregiving journey can find useful and practical advice on how to proceed at each step. It's not an exact science, but there are do's and don'ts, and knowing them will make a difference.

You can't expect to do the best for your loved one if you don't take care of yourself. Caregivers often feel isolated and in desperate need of reliable information, and there's a plethora of misinformation and well-meaning but inadequate advice available online. If you are already in the middle of this storm, you will find information here to help you put your financial and legal situation back on track.

Taking care of a patient with dementia isn't cheap, and it can bring significant financial pressure. Having stable finances can enhance the life of your loved one. Medical bills and caregiving supplies may drain your finances, and your own life may suffer. Dementia caregivers may have to reduce work hours and may not have enough energy to take care of their tasks. In some cases, they must quit a job they love and start a new job working from home to be able to take care of their loved ones.

It's not easy to distance yourself emotionally from the person you're looking after, but it helps to be practical. Knowing which documents to sign, where to apply your money, and when to say *no* will make a difference in this journey. Unless you're well-secured financially you may have to cut expenses and manage your resources. That could mean you're not always purchasing the best equipment or taking your loved one to the best doctor available. This is a balancing act between what is best and what is affordable.

Each case is different, and you need to create a personalized budget tailored to the specific needs of your loved one, which will keep you from generating future debts that you can't afford. In this book, I will guide you through identifying and accessing financial assistance programs and understanding how to leverage them effectively. We'll also discuss expense tracking and management, implementing systems for monitoring and managing ongoing expenses relative to care.

Balancing the time-intensive demands of caring for a loved one with your own personal needs, careers, and family responsibilities can lead to stress and potential burnout. I want you to know that you are not alone and that it's okay to feel lost at first. The fact that you are reading this book means you are not afraid to look for help, and that's more than most people do. The sooner you start picking yourself up and learning about your new responsibilities, the better.

One purpose of this book is to introduce you to technologies that can help you. Technology is your friend in this journey. Selecting the right technological tools that suit the needs of the person with dementia and the caregiver will put you ahead of the game. The internet will allow you to connect to other caregivers and to professionals who can give you direction. A lot of paperwork can be done through the internet these days which doesn't require you to print, fill out, and mail forms.

You can also use other technology, such as GPS tracking devices, health monitoring apps, and smart home devices, to track the health and well-being of your loved one as part of your daily routine. You might already be familiar with some of these tools without knowing how they can be applied in your situation. We will discuss that in detail and see how you can adapt to these technologies in a way that feels natural.

Caregiving is also about knowing how to navigate the minefield of legal matters that can turn your life into a nightmare. Not everyone has the required knowledge or legal experience to deal with all the directives, and it can be overwhelming to make critical legal decisions while ensuring the best interests of their loved ones are protected. Bureaucracy has the power to rustle even the most harmonious families. It can also be problematic if the caregiver makes a bad legal decision simply because they may not have known other options.

While no book can teach you all you need to know, you will learn about wills, powers of attorney, advanced directives, and other document preparation involved in caregiving. I also endeavor to enlighten you on the pathways to guardianship or conservatorship and how to interact with legal professionals. You will gain an understanding of strategies for asset protection and stay informed about legal rights and recent changes in the law.

The knowledge in this book came from my own experience as a caregiver. It wasn't easy to figure all of this out, and I wish I'd had someone to guide me through it at the time. I wrote a deeply personal book that can be used by different people. The idea isn't just to take the reader by the hand and be supportive, but instead to show how to make the best out of this experience.

As you follow this method, you will gain control of the situation and be one step ahead. Dementia is an unpredictable condition, but you can master the tools to deal with it. Even if you can't predict when your loved one is going to need a certain type of care, you can have everything ready when that happens. And even if you are not a lawyer by trade, you can understand the nuances of each legal matter that comes along.

There's a dramatic tendency to look at caregivers as martyrs— people who have abandoned their hopes and dreams dive in to a battle that can't be won. If, by the end of that battle, they are still able to stand up, they will try to pick up their lives from where they left them.

I suggest that you instead look at yourself as a strategist, someone who may not know what the next step is but who does know the best way of taking it. This way, you will be able to do a better job watching out for your loved one but also keeping yourself together. You don't have to wait for the end of this journey to start looking out for yourself. There's nothing wrong with prioritizing your own needs.

If, by the end of this book, you can make your journey less stressful and more sustainable, allowing for a quality of life that benefits both you as the caregiver and your loved one with dementia, I will have fulfilled my mission. The world changes at a fast pace, with technology taking a larger role in our lives every day. Instead of fighting those changes, we need to adapt and learn the best way of using them. Caregiving isn't the same as it was a few decades or even a few years or months ago. I propose we look at the future and see what lies ahead.

GIFT OFFER

Dear Friend,

I want to thank you so much for choosing this book, and I hope you will find it informative and supportive, but most of all compassionate. In hopes of enhancing your navigation, I am offering some complementary items that I think you will find valuable in your care journey. In addition, I would like to send you a periodic newsletter that I hope you will find helpful.

To receive your free gifts, scan the QR code using your phone or tablet, or enter the link in your browser.

CompassionateCare.fyi/get-my-gifts

Please enjoy the book!

Thank you,

L.E. Summers

BUILDING A BUDGET—
FINANCIAL LONGEVITY IN CARE

To care for those who once cared for us is one of life's highest honors. –
Tia Walker

irst, we must try to gain a comprehensive understanding of the financial implications of dementia care and get to know practical budgeting strategies that evolve with your loved one's needs. Keep in mind that these costs change with time due to the evolution of your loved one's condition, but also because healthcare is in continuous change.

Checking your loved one into a 24-hour home for seniors with dementia is a serious decision. There, they will be provided with housing, meals, medication, and activities, but they will also be away from their families for times. You should expect the home to have a safe environment designed to offer special care that includes memory-enhancing therapies and socialization with other seniors. Comprehensive support includes assistance with the following:

- housekeeping
- dressing/undressing

- incontinence care
- mobility assistance to/from common areas
- nutritious mealtimes
- laundry and linen changes
- emergency monitoring
- medication management
- memory care activities
- transportation services
- and more

Not everyone is emotionally and financially prepared to check their loved ones in a specialized care home. These facilities have highly trained staff who need to be well-paid, which increases the monthly rates. Davis (2023) calculates that the average cost of memory care in a specialized facility is around $4,635 per month, ranging up to $9,305 per month.

It helps if you can get your loved one a roommate, preferably someone who they've known for some time, and split the costs with their families. If that isn't possible, or if you've made a conscious decision to take care of your loved one yourself, it's time to learn the best way of doing that.

PREPARING FOR DEMENTIA CARE

There's a lot about caregiving that you'll have to learn during the journey, but there's also a lot you can plan for in advance. Find a professional financial planner who understands your situation and put together a strategy for your long-term costs. You can involve your loved one at this stage if they are still in the early stages of dementia and don't yet need around-the-clock care. By the time they get there, you'll already have an idea of what you face.

Getting involved in your community will also guarantee you have their assistance in moments of distress. Know your neighbors and your neighborhood. Speak openly to the people around you about the issues you're dealing with, and let them know how they can help you. Find out where all the nearest hospitals are and how you can get to them. Knowing this will make things easier in a time of distress.

You don't want to isolate your loved one; it's better to always have someone you trust by their side. Sometimes, all it takes is a simple unattended phone call for them to be caught in a scam or sign up for something unnecessary without your knowledge. During a trip to a store, they may pay ten times the value of a product because they are confused about the amount due.

Unless you're well-secured financially, you will have limited resources on this journey. Don't overlook the importance of budgeting and planning. Otherwise, you could become unable to assist your loved one at the time they need it the most. A payment that you don't make on time can escalate into a mountain of interest or the cancellation of a vital service, such as gas or electric service. Organizing your bills, paying them on time, and keeping the receipts in a safe place will save you a lot of headaches. It's helpful to automate the payments, but always keep an eye on each transaction.

People with dementia have trouble remembering their card's personal identification numbers (PINs) and online passwords. Due to the personal nature of these codes, sharing them with the entire family isn't the best choice. The caregiver should have access to them and be able to show through bank statements and other documents that they are not abusing that trust. Chip and signature cards are a good option for people with dementia since they don't require the user to memorize numbers. They are a benefit to control unwanted expenditures, as well.

There are special public services dedicated to offering financial advice to elderly people. These services are available through a phone call, such as Eldercare Locator (1-800-677-1116) and Financial Planning Association (1-800-322-4237). Another important service is the National Academy of Elder Law Attorneys, which can be reached online at naela.org.

When you look at everything that memory care involves, you may feel that you've already lost this battle. Most people can't afford the high prices of a specialized care home. Also, it's not easy to abandon your regular life to offer your loved one full-time care. Some families will unite and face this hardship together, but others will leave everything to one person—which might be you.

Cobb (2022) makes a distinction between Assisted Living Residencies (also known as memory care residences, dementia care facilities, or Alzheimer's care units), which are specially equipped to deal with patients with dementia, and nursing homes, which host senior citizens but are not specialized in dementia. In the former case, assisted living costs can range from $2,844 to $9,266/month. A regular nursing home can cost from $245/day or $7,441/month, with state daily averages ranging from $153 to $963.

Cobb (2022) also cites adult daycare centers, like a children's daycare, in which the responsible party picks them up and takes them home at the end of the day. This kind of center is not advisable to take care of people in later stages of dementia.

FINANCIAL ASSISTANCE AND ACCESS PROCEDURES

If you can't afford private health insurance, you can get assistance from Medicare, which, like most insurance, doesn't differentiate dementia from other diseases. They can help you with 100% of the specialized care home fees for 20 days, which can be extended to 80% for the following 80 days. Still, they don't pay for in-home assistance unless it's medically determined that the patient is within the last six months of their life. Private health insurance companies offer Medicare Supplement Insurance (Medigap), an extra insurance that doesn't cover dementia but can help you pay the extra 20% fees of specialized care homes that Medicare doesn't cover.

If your loved one with dementia is a U.S. veteran they can get help from Veterans Administration. Aid and Attendance Benefit which offers up to $2,500 per month of financial assistance for those who meet their criteria. There's also VA Respite Care, a program that helps pay for in-home care for veterans.

When looking for assistance, you're advised to apply for Medicaid. It can be hard to qualify, and you might need the help of an attorney. Excluding their home and typically a car, the beneficiary must exhaust all their savings before Medicaid will pay all of their care expenses.

It's possible to get employer benefits such as health savings benefits (HSA), a pre-tax savings account designed to cover qualified medical expenses by setting aside money. Some employers offer a flexible spending account (FSA) with which you can pay for medical and dental expenses for your dependent.

A reverse mortgage is another option, available to people aged 62 or older, that can convert the equity of your home into liquid funds without losing the ownership of the home. The main eligibility factors are the age, the lender's interest rate, and the home's equity. With a reverse mortgage, you can keep the benefits of your Social Security and Medicare programs, but it has an impact on applications for other government programs. You must own your home outright or pay off any existing mortgage with part of the funds from the close of the reverse mortgage.

Contact an eldercare attorney about the downsides of reverse mortgages.

As a caregiver, you can use the value of your own home to pay for the person you're assisting through a caregiver mortgage. You will have financial support for being caregivers, and your home will be protected from Medicaid estate recovery and inheritance taxes. There are different types of caregiver mortgages, such as family-funded reverse mortgages, caregiver contracts, and personal care agreements. It can be complicated to apply for them, and it's important to get professional advice before you sign anything.

You can get special loans to help you with your caregiving costs. These loans are easier to get in cases of immediate need, such as moving your loved one to a specialized care home or helping with living residence needs. As bridge loans, they are made for time periods of up to two years and can serve to cover costs while you apply for government funds. If, for example, you can't wait for the government to approve your Medicare before buying a specific medication, these loans can get you covered.

A person with dementia doesn't have to wait for the retirement age to get their retirement benefits, whether the program is personal or employee-funded. Withdrawals are typically taken after retirement. The owner of the benefits decides what an emergency is. They can use it as they wish but may incur financial penalties for early withdrawal. A dementia patient is typically retired via age or disability, and income taxes due will probably be lower as the person may fall into a lower tax bracket. Social Security benefits can also be accessed before retirement age if the individual meets the requirements for Social Security Disability Insurance (SSDI).

The National Family Caregiver Support Program (NFCSP) is an important ally for those who need support in their caregiving journey. Funded in 2000 by the Administration on Aging (AoA) of the U.S. Department of Health and Human Services, the NFCSP offers special grants and assistance to caregivers, shares information, and offers respite care and supplemental services on a limited basis. Their aim isn't just to help people financially but also to help with depression, anxiety, and stress that affect caregivers. Informal caregivers of patients with Alzheimer's and other forms of dementia are eligible to receive the services of the NFCSP. They also help the elderly who are taking care of children and younger relatives with disabilities. *Contact* the Area Agency on Aging in your area either by calling 1-800-994-9422 or by visiting their website at acl.gov.

Social Security offers a program known as the Compassionate Allowance Program, which you can engage in by submitting a form to the Supplement Security Administration. Aimed at those retired by age, they offer allowances for memory care for disabilities, including dementia diagnosis. When the diagnosis happens before retirement, you can apply for Social Security Disability Insurance (SSDI).

The Alzheimer's Disease Programs Initiative (ADPI) is an organization dedicated to uniting caregivers around the US, addressing their needs, and offering grants and activities in partnership with the National Alzheimer's and Dementia Resource Center (NADRC). Never losing sight of the human element, the ADPI aims to implement evidence-based supportive services for patients with dementia and their caregivers. They also collaborate with public and private entities to meet the needs of patients and their families.

Available 24 hours a day, seven days a week, 365 days a year, at 1-800-272-3900, the National Alzheimer's Call Center works in all 50 states, and most U.S. territories. By calling it, you will be put in touch with an expert who can offer you free advice and consultation and direct you where to look for help. Their staff is composed of social workers with advanced training and proven experience as social workers. They may not have all the answers that you need at the moment, but they will tell you the best place to look for assistance, whether your local Alzheimer's Association chapter or another organization in your area.

FINANCIAL MANAGING AND COMMON PITFALLS

Difficulties in managing their own money is one of the key signs that a person may be suffering from dementia when they have been successfully managing perfectly fine in the past. This is a consequence of their limited cognitive abilities and memory issues, which can make them spend too much or put their money in the wrong places. Patients with dementia also have a harder time remembering to pay for their credit cards and pay for rent, utilities, and medical bills.

When your loved one is diagnosed with some form of dementia, you might feel the urge to act as fast as possible. With the clock ticking, you want to put everything into place before the condition gets worse. Still, it's important to be calm and calculate each step of the way to prevent further trouble.

Whether you're taking them to a specialized care home or planning to act as a caregiver, you may expect money problems later. Wong (2023) states that: "From 2004 to 2020, the cost for a nursing home facility has increased from 1.88%–3.80% per year." Things got worse with the COVID-19 pandemic when staff had to adopt special health and safety measures.

While managing another person's money it's wise to start with an inventory. You need to gather all the documentation to know where that person's money is and what kind of document they may have signed in the past; get their bank account and credit card statements, insurance policies, trust documents, mortgages, and loans. You need to be clear about all their debts and income so you can start putting together a plan.

With all of that in hand, it's time to prepare a bill payment schedule, knowing where the money comes from and where it's supposed to go. In some cases, the money will come from the patient, but members of the family may also contribute with their own money. Whatever the case is, it's important to pay for everything at the right time. That means that anyone who wants to contribute must do so punctually.

If you don't have a printer with a scanner or a photocopier, it's time to get one. You need records of all the documentation that passes through your hands, from medical equipment to the soda you got at the hospital's machine. This is important not only for tax purposes but also when family members start arguing that you're spending too much.

Organize a family meeting to talk about these plans. As the caregiver, you should have primary access to the caregiving funds in case you need them for an emergency. Other family members may have access to it to help you pay the bills, arrange benefit claims, and prepare tax returns, among others. Everyone can avoid trouble by being as transparent as possible about this process.

Soon after a diagnosis, it is important to talk about finances and future care wishes. Start by collecting and organizing important documents. Seek help from well-qualified financial and legal advisors and estimate the possible costs for the entire disease process. There are many insurance options that serve different kinds of work-related salary/benefits. Find out which government programs you are eligible for and learn about income tax breaks that you may qualify for through the patient's benefits or their spouse's. Apart from financial assistance, there are also free or low-cost community services that can serve your needs.

It's time to tailor a budget plan based on your situation. Below, you will find some of the most important points that you will have to address as an in-home dementia caregiver.

Average Monthly Expenses for In-Home Dementia Care

Agency vs. Independent Caregiver

Caregivers may be working by themselves or for agencies. Independent caregivers are slightly less costly, but they are not as reliable. In case of an emergency, an agency can send a different caregiver to replace the official one, which doesn't happen with independent caregivers. The process of hiring an independent caregiver also requires more effort.

Care Needs Level

As your loved one's condition progresses, their needs will change. While it's hard to plan for that in advance, it helps to keep resources available as things progress. If, for example, they start having trouble walking, it helps to have set apart money to buy a walker or scooter.

Home Modifications

The price of home modifications is different in each case. You can find items such as grab bars at a wide range of different prices, and different types will serve different needs. The price of installation also varies, and it's better not to go too cheap, or you could have problems with their function.

Products for Dementia Patients

You can find products specially designed for the elderly, many of which are created specifically for patients with dementia. From house alarms to special beds, these products vary in price and quality. You need to consider these two factors while making your purchase, taking into account your money limitations and the necessities of your loved one.

SEGUE

As we end this introductory chapter, I hope you are aware of what's coming and the importance of considering every detail. Having a loved one with dementia is such an overwhelming process that we tend to forget the most practical aspects of it. This is an uphill battle, and there will be sleepless nights and moments of distress. You can alleviate a good deal of those moments if you have your paperwork in place and bills paid.

We have seen the importance of choosing the right legal and healthcare options. You need to go through them carefully and select the best option for you and your loved one. Find out what suits you, and don't be afraid to ask questions. You can find other people who are or have been in the same situation as you, but the most sound advice will always come from a trained professional who knows what they're doing.

Money can be a complicated matter, as any Wall Street executive will tell you, and it's not different with healthcare and insurance. Signing any document without reading the fine print can jeopardize your future well-being. You can't expect to know all about the matter, and it helps to get legal help in these situations. But it's also crucial that you know enough about it yourself so you can make fast decisions during complicated situations.

Now that you know how to put together a sustainable budget, we have set the cornerstone of our journey. It's time to start building a sustainable financial edifice that will endure against potential healthcare storms. Insurance options and processes are a complicated matter, and you need to be prepared for what lies ahead. So, let's dive into it!

2

ASSESS THE CARE NEEDS OF YOUR LOVED ONE

To be prepared is half the victory. –Miguel de Cervantes

*a*s you navigate through the many dementia healthcare options, you might feel lost in an ocean of names and numbers. My goal with this chapter is to give you a comprehensive understanding of long-term care insurance options tailored for dementia care, including the intricacies of long-term care insurance, Medicare, and Medicaid, which we've already mentioned.

As the responsible party for a patient with dementia, you can't afford to learn things by trial and error. Instead, you must know what works for you, how to make it work, and, just as important, what you shouldn't even try. By the end of the chapter, these application processes won't feel as mysterious, and you will be able to address common issues related to them.

NAVIGATING INSURANCE OPTIONS

As a progressive disease, dementia shows itself little by little. Signs start to appear related to a person's daily activities and self-care until the moment they start to worry the family. By then, the family should start looking for medical help, including long-term care professionals. Paying for long-term care can drain a family's savings, but it's possible to apply for programs such as the ones we discussed in the previous chapter.

Finding the right type of insurance policy isn't easy. Brokers must make sales and might try to push you into something that doesn't offer what you need, so get a second opinion. A good place to start is with long-term care insurance or LTC insurance. These cover medical services that may help with basic functions. Long-term insurance can be traditional, meaning it contains a specific policy that covers one's expenses for long-term care. It can also be hybrid, meaning that they are paid together with other kinds of policies, including life insurance and funeral plans.

Memory care provides specialized staff that can help patients with dementia. They are trained to maintain quality of life while also assisting the patient in their daily lives. With this type of policy, you can expect your loved one to be fed, bathed, cleaned, and medicated, while also keeping in touch with the community, doing stimulating activities such as memory games and physical activities, having assistance with mobility, and getting physical and occupational therapies.

It sounds amazing, but not everyone gets approved for long-term care insurance. The family is advised to apply for that kind of insurance for your loved one when dementia hasn't settled yet, around the age of 50-65. If the individual already has dementia or needs other kinds of long-term care services, it can be harder to get approved. Insurance companies conduct a battery of tests to determine if the person has mitigating circumstances or has cognitive impairments that keep them from learning, reasoning, paying attention, or making decisions.

The policy will specify the date on which the coverage begins. Even then, there's often a waiting line called the elimination period. This can go from one to three months, and the family might have to bear the costs of the dementia treatment during this period, which may be reimbursed by the insurance later on. Long-term care insurance often has an optional rider known as inflation protection to cope with rising care costs.

Never sign an insurance policy without being sure of its maximum daily benefit, how its costs adjust to inflation, and what kind of reimbursement you may be entitled to. Be as rigorous with them as they are with you. Figure out the amount of each coverage and how the patient can qualify for coverage if they already have health problems. Each long-term policy is tailored to different circumstances, and you shouldn't compare your situation with someone else's.

According to the National Council on Aging (*Medicare*, 2023), for each $900 paid annually, a 55-year-old man in 2023 can expect to get $165,000 worth of coverage. A woman of the same age would pay $1,500 annually to get the same coverage.

To get the ideal policy, you need to assess the care needs of your loved one. Knowing the stage of your loved one's dementia will help you to select the best possible insurance policy. Avoid exaggeration or trying to make things sound worse than they are to get more robust coverage. That can backfire and instead make you lose the coverage altogether.

Finding long-term care insurance covering dementia care costs isn't difficult, but not all of them are equipped to deal with all cases. There's also the matter of when to start. We mentioned that you should start a policy for your loved one before they get dementia. The problem is, you could be paying for a long time before you need it, in which case the costs could become unbearable. You may also continue to pay for the rest of your loved ones' lives without them developing dementia.

The right long-term care insurance will provide your loved one with doctor's appointments and prescription medications. They should also get them physical and occupational therapy and medical equipment—wheelchairs and walkers, for example.

Long-term care policies are still available, with many now being linked to life insurance policies. The death benefit is paid when other benefits remain without use for a long time. Over time, these policies accumulate value, allowing for a partial return of the amount paid if surrendered. Typically, premiums are paid for a fixed number of years, after which the policy is considered "paid up." It's important to note that there may be other variations of long-term care insurance as this method of insuring against specific risks continues to evolve. Those who can't afford the costs above and beyond Medicare can apply to several programs operated by Medicaid itself. Ask for more information at the time of your application.

Read each policy carefully to make sure that you are not signing into something that could harm you or your loved one down the road. Today's insurance policies are written in clear language, but if you feel that the language of the insurance policy is too technical or if you are not getting the answers you need, it's wise to seek the assistance of a legal professional.

You should get what you pay for and know what provisions you're entitled to. To get that, you will need a licensed health-care professional to conduct exams on your loved one to prove that they need assistance to perform their daily activities and that they have cognitive impairment. Through that examination, the insurance company will determine the needs of your loved one. They will make sure that the people taking care of your loved one are licensed healthcare practitioners, such as nurses, physicians, and social workers. Policies should contain a detailed description of each activity and the necessity of improving them over time.

Medicare provides coverage for up to 100 days of care in a skilled nursing facility (SNF) for each benefit period. For more than 100 days of SNF care within a benefit period, the patient will have to pay the costs. Medicare also offers physical, occupational, or speech therapy, and it's possible to continue getting coverage for this kind of skilled therapy services even after exhausting your benefit.

Hospital and skilled nursing care may be covered by Medicare A, while doctor services, home health care, outpatient care, and durable medical equipment are covered by Medicare B. For Medicare B, you need to pay a fee each month. The current fee for 2024 is $174.70, while those with a modified adjusted income must pay extra.

Medicare B requires a monthly premium, which leads some people to delay their application. The dementia patient often shares group health insurance with their spouse or gets it through their employer. After losing that coverage, you need to apply for Medicare B within eight months, under the risk of penalties. You will need to complete Form CMS-40B (Application for Enrollment in Medicare–Part B) and, in some cases, Form CMS-L564 (Request for Employment Information) if you want to request a special enrollment period.

Medicare covers an annual wellness visit, in which the doctor or health professional requests a Medicare beneficiary (or caregiver) to complete a health risk assessment (HRA). This assessment provides valuable information and serves improve the diagnostic process. Care partners or caregivers can share information with the physician before the Annual Wellness Visit to ensure a comprehensive assessment.

Individuals who have recently been diagnosed with dementia can benefit from Medicare's care planning services. They teach patients and their caregivers about medical and non-medical treatments, community services, clinical trials, and other resources that can enhance their quality of life. You will find information about it here, but you are *always* advised to consult an insurance professional before taking any further steps.

Medicare C is also known as Medicare Advantage, and it offers different options for managed care, such as preferred provider organization (PPO), point of service (POS), and Medicare health maintenance organization (HMO). Each of them offers different features, and again, you should read each policy with care before signing. Medicare also offers special needs plans (SNPs) for individuals with dementia, providing specialized care and coverage for Medicare beneficiaries suffering from dementia.

STEP-BY-STEP PROCESS FOR MEDICARE AND MEDICAID APPLICATIONS

Applying to Medicare online is a straightforward process, taking from 10 to 15 minutes. People who already receive benefits from Social Security don't have to apply again. If that's not the case, you have a seven-month window to apply, which starts three months before and ends three months after your birthdate. Within this window, you can apply for Medicare Part A and B online or through fax or mail. You can also show up at your local Social Security office and apply in person. To be eligible for Part B, you need to already be enrolled in Part A.

Once you enter your data, your application will be processed, and you will get a red, white, and blue Medicare card within two to three months. The card will have the enrollee's name, Medicare beneficiary identifier number, and the start dates for Medicare A and B coverage.

To avoid penalties for not signing up at 65, you must complete and submit two forms (CMS 40B and CMS-L564) to Social Security. These forms demonstrate your coverage under employer or other creditable insurance. If you can provide proof of coverage, you won't face any penalties.

The initial online application for Medicare can be completed by visiting ssa.gov or socialsecurity.gov. They require you to create an account if you don't have one, with a username and a password. Once you set up your account, follow these steps:

- On the ssa.gov home page, click on Medicare enrollment.
- Scroll down until you find the blue button that says, "Apply to Medicare Only".
- By clicking on the button, you'll be redirected to terms of service.
- Check the box stating that you understand and agree with their terms, and click next.
- Here, you can start an application, offering the requested information:
- Do you want to apply for Medicare only or with Social Security?
- Do you want to apply for full benefits for Parts A and B?
- Do you already have any insurance coverage, and if so, what are the start and end dates?

At the end of this process, they'll give you a confirmation link through which you can consult your application. Save this link and have it at hand to consult it whenever you need. For most people, the only eligibility criteria to apply to Medicare is being 65. You may also be able to apply if you're a railroad worker and are part of the Railroad Retirement Board.

Have the following documents at hand:

- a copy of the applicant's birth certificate
- an I.D. card or driver's license
- Social Security card
- a document proving you're a U.S. citizen
- medical information

Apart from the website, you can also call Social Security at 1-800-772-1213 (TTY 1-800-325-0778), 7 a.m. to 7 p.m., Monday through Friday.

Once you enroll in Medicare, it's time to create an account on MyMedicare.gov so you can manage your online coverage. There, you'll be able to update our information, get details about your plans, enter new records, view your claims, print cards, and get in touch with providers. You can do this by accessing www.medicare.gov/account/create-account and entering the information found on your red, white, and blue card.

You may consider applying for Medicare C (Medicare Advantage), which offers the same benefits found in the two other parts, plus prescription drug coverage and dental and vision treatment.

Each person who applies for Medicare must go through a process that's specific to their needs. In most cases, you'll get a card three weeks after your application. Those who are already enrolled can expect to get their card in the mail two months before they turn 65. If you don't receive your decision notification on time or have your application denied, it's possible to appeal through a state fair hearing.

Medigap, also referred to as optional supplemental insurance policies, assists in covering deductible costs, out-of-pocket copays, and coinsurance expenses that are not covered by

Medicare. To be eligible to enroll in Medigap, you must first be enrolled in Medicare Part A and Part. To apply to Medigap:

- go to the Medicare website
- look for Medigap finder
- enter your zip code
- offer the required information plans
- review the costs
- choose a plan and click View Policies
- identify the right policy and make an application

The website offers the option of connecting with the policy companies to get more information as needed.

INTERACTIVE ELEMENT

Here are the four types of health insurance plans according to the website HealthCare.gov:

- The **Bronze Plan** is tailored for those who want to be covered in an extreme case, such as a serious disease or injury. It won't do much for those looking for routine care.
- The **Silver Plan** is more suited for those looking for routine care treatment and is only a little more expensive than Bronze.
- The **Gold Plan** covers more routine costs and is suited for those who need constant medical care.
- The **Platinum Plan** is for those who can afford to pay a higher amount each month to cover all sorts of medical treatment, from emergencies to daily care.

Keep in mind that the situation with your loved one may change, and you might have to migrate to a different kind of plan. This isn't always an easy process if you can't afford it, but it's best to know how it works.

SEGUE

Dealing with insurance can be a nightmare, but you must know what you're doing before signing on. There are many options out there, and for the healthcare companies profit is their main goal. Still, you can find one that suits your needs and will be there for you at your moment of need. We've seen how to apply to Medicare, with all its nuances, giving you a better grasp of the insurance options and how to navigate them.

You're now prepared to face the legal aspects of caregiving with confidence. In the next chapter, we'll discover the financial aspects and tools you'll need to secure the well-being of your loved one and ensure your peace of mind.

3

SAFEGUARDING ASSETS

The greatest legacy one can pass on to one's children and grandchildren is not money or other material things accumulated in one's life, but rather a legacy of character and faith. —Billy Graham

It's now time to master the strategies for preserving the financial legacy of their loved ones with dementia. Making sure that your loved one won't run out of money is as important as preventing them from falling in the shower or getting their medicine on time.

Even if you're used to taking care of your own finances, there's still a lot to learn about how to manage the assets of a person with dementia. Knowing where each cent is and where it's supposed to go will prevent you from being caught off guard in life-or-death situations. At the end of this chapter, you should feel equipped with the tools and understanding necessary to safeguard assets and secure the financial support needed for long-term care.

STRATEGIES FOR PLANNING

Staying at a hospital can be distressing for a patient with dementia, and most of them prefer the familiarity of their own home. Mitchell et al. (2012) affirm that the future of dementia treatment lies in offering high-quality treatment in different settings that take into account the patient's background in a place they can call their own, which will help them to remain active and healthy while also coping with memory loss.

It's important that you take action fast after a dementia diagnosis. Introduce the subject to your family members, prioritizing practical actions. Important documents, such as medical records, should be secured in one place and regularly updated as the situation develops. One person should be ensured with those documents, but it's wise to create copies for emergencies. Family members need to be in contact with doctors and lawyers, always granting the caregiver the power to make important decisions.

The Alzheimer's Association lists the following documents that need to be gathered ("Making Financial Plans After a Diagnosis of Dementia," 2016):

Legal documents:

- living wills
- medical and durable powers of attorney
- wills
- bank and brokerage account information
- deeds, mortgage papers, or ownership statements
- insurance policies
- outstanding bills (monthly, quarterly, or annually)
- pension and retirement benefit summaries
- Social Security payment information
- stock and bond certificates

- other sources of monthly income, e.g., rental property, sale of stocks, interest

With those in hand, you can start planning for expenses in the short, middle, and long term. Spend as much time as you feel you need with doctors, getting to know the treatment your loved one will be going through. This way, you can plan for future medical expenses as medications change and as the costs of professional help from nurses and caregivers increase regularly.

Finding or being the best possible caregiver is a continuous struggle. When dementia is part of your reality, the last thing you want is to deal with unprepared people who may do more harm than good. Being a professional caregiver is an inglorious task since this is a physically and psychologically demanding profession that's often underpaid. High-quality training is available for caregivers, but not every patient can afford it. You might choose to invest in your caregiver, paying for them to get better training, or get that training yourself for when you have to deal with your loved one on your own.

It's important to understand the concept of financial capacity, which means the ability to manage your financial matters in a way that's consistent with your self-interest and your values. It doesn't mean just having money to fulfill your daily needs, but being mentally able to manage those costs and others that may arise. That can be a problem for patients with dementia and other diseases that affect cognition, such as stroke, traumatic brain injury, and schizophrenia, as well as neurodegenerative conditions like Alzheimer's.

Financial capacity is a worrying matter for family members of patients with dementia. They may be afraid that their loved one will make damaging financial choices and be misguided by people who want to take advantage of them. They may also offer gifts that don't fit their financial situation and have trouble creating a fair will, leading to disputes inside the family.

Financial capacity doesn't get as much clinical and ethical consideration as it should in dementia scientific literature. However, it plays a huge role in the well-being of patients and their families. It gives independence to the patient, prevents awkward situations in their daily lives, and protects them against scammers.

Research conducted by Li et al. (2022) states that: "In 2018, 7.4 million older US adults with dementia or CIND [Cognitive impairment with no dementia] were managing their household finances". Due to their cognitive problems, these people often mismanaged their money. The study shows that elderly people who could count on the involvement of their families in their finances had more success in managing their assets. Another study by Sturge et al. (2021) states that to improve the well-being of people with memory problems such as dementia, it's important to have the community's support.

Without proper planning, the cost of caring for a patient with dementia can leave you in a worrying financial state. Most of that has to do with medical costs, but there's also the fact that people with dementia tend to make bad financial decisions. This includes credit card debt, unpaid taxes, loans, and the simple act of lending money that is never paid back.

One solution is to add dementia costs to your loved one's health plan even before they show signs of it. Nobody wants to imagine their father having dementia, but it doesn't hurt to be cautious. That can teach you a lot about how you're spending your finances at the moment and make you more cautious about the future.

Being a caregiver for a loved one is a hard, tough, and perhaps unpaid job, and it can become unbearable if you don't have a structure around you. Part of that structure consists of families and other loved ones who may assist you with services and money. But you also need to have a financial and psychological structure that will give you security and independence to fulfill these tasks.

Being a caregiver will affect your career and your social life, and it can last for several years. It's important to be prepared from the beginning. Getting the help of a professional financial advisor can make a difference at this point. Financial advisors need to be money specialists or investment consultants—they need to able to be humane and careful as they take you through the necessary steps.

A patient's autonomy relies on their capacity to make decisions through an assessment of risks and benefits. As dementia progresses, the patient with dementia will need someone else to make those decisions for them. This makes them more vulnerable and can affect their right to dignity. It's a mistake to think that the dementia diagnosis eliminates a person's autonomy, but financial decision-making abilities are often the first ones to decline. This causes a problem, for the people dealing with the dementia patient's money may abuse this power and use the money for their purposes.

People with dementia are vulnerable to scammers. Through a phone call or email, someone can make up a story and ask for personal details, such as ID and credit card number. Even a legit company, such as a bank, can sell a service to a person with dementia, offering something they don't need, and that will leave them financially crippled. Banks and credit card companies often have fraud alerts that you can activate to prevent get-rich-quick offers, scams, or even threats for money.

With basic math skills and some common sense, it's possible to make basic wise financial choices. To go further than that, it's important to keep detailed records of each place where you spent money, including philanthropic donations. The enemy might be closer than that.

None of this is new for the legal system, which offers some remedies for this kind of situation. It's worse when the family doesn't have a common accord about who's going to be the caregiver. This is the person who's going to manage the assets of the patient with dementia, and all must agree they're trustworthy.

A guardianship can be established by the members of the family in common accord. It can also be made legal by submitting an evaluation to a judge, but that process can be long, expensive, and stressful. Evaluations are often intrusive and traumatic for everyone involved, and even then, the chosen guardian may not live up to their commitment.

While it's important to gather the family during the early stages of dementia to discuss the financial plan, their participation shouldn't end there. The ideal thing is to have regular meetings to discuss the budget and the management of the bills, plan for long-term care costs, and make sure that everyone has access to the paperwork involved. This guarantees transparency and can prevent future feuds.

DEFINING STRATEGIES

Whatever strategies you decide to take, take them as soon as possible after the dementia diagnosis. Everyone needs to be prepared for what's to come, and knowing the next steps will make a difference. Be aware that plans will change as the condition progresses, but that doesn't take away the importance of careful preparation.

You might want to set up a fund to cover all your loved one's expenses, medical or otherwise. Not every family member will be able to contribute the same amount of money to that fund. Still, everyone who takes part in it should have an equal voice in each decision. Be careful with how much direct access your loved one with dementia gets to that fund—depending on the stage of their condition, as they could be easy targets for fraud and scams.

Dialogue is key in this project. Family and friends need to be transparent about their role in this process, defining what each one can and cannot do. They all have to participate in the creation of the budget, for that will make it more efficient. Setting automated bill payments is a good way of making sure everything is paid at the right time, and everyone knows where the money is coming from and where it's going.

The budget should be tight, with no space for unnecessary purchases. The needs of the loved one with dementia should be put above everything else. Family members shouldn't be allowed to borrow or spend this money to satisfy their own needs.

There will be unexpected expenses, such as new medicines, equipment, or health services, that need to be accounted for. You might also have to add long-term costs, such as assisted living, a nursing home, or surgery. The entire family should be aware of what's going on. There's always a chance someone won't be happy with those expenses, but again, you have to prioritize the patient's needs.

With the progression of the disease, you might have to assume control over your loved one's financial affairs. Take action while they're still able to understand legal arrangements, and take them to a lawyer who can arrange a power of attorney—a document that gives legal authority for you to act on your loved one's behalf as they lose their mental capacity.

ETHICS OF CAREGIVING

A caregiver needs to practice beneficence, which is a fancy word for doing the right thing. That means being kind to the person you're looking after and not doing them harm. This involves all of your interactions, from answering the same question several times to being gentle as you bathe them. Beneficence is a simple concept that needs to be acknowledged if you want the best for your loved one.

The dementia patient still has the right to be empowered and make decisions regarding their condition and treatment. As a caregiver, your role is to act in the best interest of the person you're caring for, even if those clash with your own. They need your support, but their personality still matters, even if they are in the late stages of the disease. Dementia patients can still surprise you with how much they're capable of. The progression of dementia isn't linear, with symptoms varying in each case, and you can't generalize their cognitive deficit.

A patient with dementia can enjoy their autonomy through their relationship with others and by sticking to their values. If, for example, they have a pet that they are very fond of, that feeling gives them the right to maintain that pet. It's not for the family to decide to get rid of it because they are making a mess in the house.

The things you know about that person from living with them before dementia will help you after they can no longer make decisions. They will respond better if you give them limited options to choose between. Instead of asking, "Do you want butter on your bread?" you can ask if they prefer butter or jelly. This makes things easier and allows them the right to choose.

As the capacity to make decisions fades, the family needs to step forward and fulfill that role. The substitute decision-maker, or makers, must know the person from before the disease, knowing their values and wishes. Those can be written down and saved in an advance directive, a document that will guide the decisions of that patient's future care.

Be careful not to start making decisions on a person's behalf while they're still capable of doing them on their own. That may happen if their wishes contradict yours or can cause harm to the person making it. It's not always easy. For example, they might insist on keeping a maid who is very nice but steals objects from the house. You need to assess the impact of firing that maid will have on your loved one's mind, in comparison to the risk of having a thief inside the house.

Having an inventory of everything in the house will serve in case something is missing. You should know everyone who's coming in and out of the house, from the caregiver to the plumber who came once to fix the shower. If someone from the family wants to take something, like a book or a DVD player, they should always let someone know when they take it and when they plan to return it.

Letting a person with dementia live alone can be a risk. Elderly people tend to prefer staying at their own house instead of moving with a relative or checking into home care. However, if they're at a stage in which they can't look after their own safety, it might be the time to look at having someone moving in with them. In that situation, most of the caregiving responsibilities will be on that person's shoulders, and they should have all the support they need from the rest of the family.

Asset protection is crucial for dementia patients. The disease can go on for a long time, and you need to secure funds for its duration. This planning should include the progression of the disease, and you need to conserve existing savings, investments, income, and real estate.

Here are some care costs to take into consideration:

- medical treatment for dementia symptoms
- medical treatment for other diseases
- medical equipment
- home safety modification
- prescription drugs
- personal care supplies
- in-home care services
- full-time residential care services

Check the ones that you've already taken care of and write down what you can do about the ones that you had not considered. While you're at it, check the list below and find out what steps to take next.

- Determine the roles of family members that may help you financially.
- Determine the roles of family members that may help you in other ways, such as offering services or providing important contacts.
- Organize all needed documents, and find out if your loved one has acquired any insurance policies in the past.
- Make an inventory of all assets and debts regarding your loved one's finances.

- Find out if you're eligible for government benefits that can help you with medication, transportation, and meals.
- If your loved one served in the army forces, they may be eligible for Veteran benefits.

SEGUE

Everyone has an opinion on whether money brings happiness. Still, it's undeniable that money can bring a lot of distress, ruin relationships, and disrupt entire families. That's true for wealthy families but also for the rest of us, which is why transparency and ethics are crucial.

In this chapter, we've seen how things can go wrong with the finances of a family dealing with the effects of dementia on a loved one. We've also learned that planning on how to use that money can save a lot of headaches. While the main caregiver should be put in charge of important decisions, the entire family should participate in this process.

Now that you have secured financial foundations, it's time to look at the legalities involved in caregiving. Knowing about the law and the kind of documents involved in elder care will make a difference when you must deal with lawyers and other legal professionals.

4

FORESIGHT IN LAW—LEGAL PREPAREDNESS

In preparing for battle I have always found that plans are useless, but planning is indispensable. –Dwight D. Eisenhower

aking the time to learn how legal documents work will give you the power to make your own decisions. You don't need a law degree to deal with important legal matters. While you should always get legal advice from a qualified professional, it helps to understand what kind of documents you're signing and which ones you shouldn't sign. It also helps to select the best possible eldercare attorney that you can afford, allowing you to work together with them instead of assuming a passive role.

In this chapter, you'll learn the steps to draft a will, establish powers of attorney, and create advance directives to protect your loved one. Additionally, you'll receive advice on selecting and collaborating with eldercare attorneys. This will empower you with legal foresight, ensuring that you are thoroughly prepared for future legalities in caring for someone with dementia.

FIND AN ELDERCARE ATTORNEY

Getting an attorney who respects you and your loved one is important. Getting a specialist in eldercare will make things go smoothly. A specialist will advise you on how to protect your assets, prepare the necessary documents, and assist the family after your loved one has passed away. The services of a reputable elder law attorney will safeguard your senior's legal and financial situation while covering necessary care. They can save your family a lot of money and prevent any future legal complications.

Since laws change between states, you may need assistance to prepare the necessary legal documents. Engaging a local eldercare attorney will ensure you complete those documents in accordance with federal, state, and local regulations.

Family or friends can refer you to a lawyer they like to work with. It's better to get a referral from someone with the same legal needs as yours or from other competent lawyers who can refer you to a colleague. If you know and trust any financial advisors, accountants, or fiduciaries, consider asking them for a referral, for these professionals often collaborate with elder law attorneys. When in doubt, consult The National Academy of Elder Law Attorneys (NAELA), which has a database of lawyers you can consult.

A lawyer specializing in eldercare will help you offer special attention to your loved one. They will be able to help in cases that involve issues such as:

- Social Security benefits
- defense of guardianship
- abuse
- neglect
- age discrimination

- protective services
- health care, including Medicare, long-term care, and nutrition
- housing, including eviction or issues with a landlord
- income security

Once you get referrals, you need to select a lawyer. Arrange a meeting to discuss your case and verify their credentials. A personal meeting will give you a sense of their working style and help you figure out if they're a good match. Most lawyers offer a complimentary 15 to 30-minute meeting, so take advantage of it. Meet multiple lawyers, compare their responses, and figure out if you like their approach.

A lawyer needs experience in cases such as yours to be a good fit. That experience is measured in years of practice. They need to be there for you, responding to calls and emails, explaining the law in simple terms, and fulfilling their promises. Before hiring an attorney, always check the State Bar Association website for your state to be sure that they have an active license to practice law.

ESSENTIAL LEGAL DOCUMENTS

The best time to get into action is during the first stages of mild dementia when you notice that your loved one has trouble remembering new information. This process goes smoother if all family members are working together to define each other's roles and put together a plan for what lies ahead. You need to be honest with each other about the difficulties that lie ahead and give priority to the well-being of the patient as well as the caregiver. This is true even in cases in which the patient is in a care facility.

At this point, when a caregiver is welcome but not essential, you should start gathering the necessary legal documents. Make sure that you get the following information regarding the finances of your loved one, as this information will be necessary in creating legal documents:

- **Assets list:** including their investment accounts, real estate, vehicles, collectibles, private business interests, annuities, and others.
- **Digital assets:** Login accounts, IDs, and passwords.
- **Important contacts:** Emails and phone numbers from people who manage their finances, such as accountants, lawyers, bankers, and health care professionals.
- **Insurance policies.**
- **Liabilities list:** recurring bills such as mortgages, credit cards, and other obligations.

It's crucial to have the names and contact data of each fiduciary registered with precise details so you can contact the right people when they're needed. This includes family members, health professionals, attorneys, business partners, and anyone interested in this process. It's also important to determine how each person fits in, giving them the proper designations.

The following documents may not already exist, in which case you should have them drawn up:

- **Health care proxy (HCP):** When your loved one is no longer able to make decisions by themselves, this document gives power to a designee to make decisions in their best interest.
- **HIPAA authorization:** This document authorizes medical professionals to inform the family members contemplated in the HCP about details in the patient's state that may influence their decisions.

- **DNR (do not resuscitate):** the living will and the advanced directive: We'll discuss these in detail in the following chapters.
- **Durable power of attorney (DPA):** Gives a specific person, usually a member of the family, the authority to manage all matters for the patient when they're no longer able to take care of their property affairs and health issues.
- **Will:** The will of a person with dementia should be reviewed by an executor to ensure that they were in sound mind as they distributed their assets.
- **Removable Trust:** Appoints a trustee who will manage the patient's assets once they're legally unable to take care of them by themselves. This includes decisions regarding how to spend money for medical care and equipment and to authorize payments for the caregiver.
- **Irrevocable trust:** Despite the name, this trust isn't unchangeable. It's a contract between the grantor (the patient), the family, and the trustee, who will control the trust and administer the situation like a business.
- **Real estate:** If the patient has any real estate assets, the ideal is to transfer them to the spouse or the revocable trust.
- **Other accounts:** From cable TV bills to magazine subscriptions and gym memberships, you need to gather information about all of your loved ones' accounts.

CREATING A WILL

Creating a will requires testamentary capacity, which means the person must understand the meaning of the document and its implications. They also must be aware of the assets they own and which people they're including in the will. This capacity can be disputed by the people contemplated in the will, and it will save you some trouble to have a doctor's report stating they have the capacity.

It's possible for anyone to do a will by themselves through digital templates that can be found online or in office supply stores. Still, considering the sensitive nature of the document, it's advisable to get professional help to make sure everything is done correctly. Without it, the terms of the will can be misinterpreted, and the deceased's wishes may not be fulfilled. Another reason to consult a specialist is that laws vary from state to state, and you will need someone who can guide you through this process.

A will requires witnesses who are not usually contemplated among the heirs. If you're doing it by yourself, you'll need to find your own. They also require executors, who are the people who will manage your estate. That person can be anyone, but it's advisable to get a professional such as an attorney or a banker. Don't confuse the executor with the power of attorney —the latter only takes care of a person's estate after their death. People included in the power of attorney should have access to the will, which can only be opened after the patient's demise. Having a successor for that power of attorney is helpful in case they or the executor of the will are unavailable to fulfill their role.

A will isn't supposed to be a flourished piece of literature. The person writing it needs to be clear and precise, offering lists of items and instructions on how to distribute them. If your loved one is leaving assets to a minor or any person who can't look after themselves, they might have to do so through a trust. Apart from physical assets, a will may also include digital ones, such as internet accounts, usernames, and passwords. Those shouldn't be informed directly on the will, which is a public document but in a private message.

The reading of the will doesn't have to be a dramatic reveal. Often, people go to those readings knowing what they will get, for it's been talked about with their loved ones. It's up to your loved one who'll be compensated in the will. They need to distribute their assets in a reasonable manner—two people who live far apart can't share the same car, for example.

People often write different wills at different stages of their lives. As times change, assets change value, relationships begin and end, and people change their minds about what they're going to leave behind. This is especially true for digital assets since passwords and logins are always changing, and platforms come and go.

A living will is a different document in which a person expresses their wishes regarding healthcare at the end of their lives. Here, they express if they want to go through surgery, resuscitation, ventilators, and feeding tubes. These wishes can be expressed in detail or in a general manner. For example, the person may not want to get surgery with a high risk of mortality while accepting one that offers lower risks.

POWER OF ATTORNEY AND GUARDIANSHIP

As dementia progresses, the caregiver is supposed to look after the patient's daily routine, such as feeding and hygiene. However, other important matters need to be addressed, especially financial issues and health preparations. During their entire life, your loved one has acquired debts and assets, made investments, and saved money for the future. Those things won't vanish because of their condition and need to be taken care of.

Once again, the first step is to gather all the papers regarding those matters. As annoying as the process of putting together this document can be, it will make things easier down the line.

Whenever possible, it's better to take care of this during the early stages of dementia to save labor for when things get more complicated. By then, having a solid power of attorney will help in the harshest decisions.

In a power of attorney, the dementia patient—referred to as the principal—appoints an individual—referred to as the agent—to make decisions on their behalf when they can't. Whether the agent is a spouse, partner, family member, or trusted friend, they need to understand how serious their responsibility is. The writing of a power of attorney should leave no room for interpretation and becomes valid when the principal loses their capacity to make decisions.

With a power of attorney for healthcare, the agent has the power to make decisions regarding medical matters. This includes the type of treatments that the patient will get, getting fed through a tube, and the decision to do not resuscitate (DNR).

A similar legal process is a guardianship, through which a guardian is designated to make important decisions for an incapacitated adult patient. This could be anyone who suffers from an incapacitating disease, including dementia. It's the guardian's job to decide the patient's health, safety, and care.

Incapacity is defined as the loss of cognitive issues that render a person unable to look after themselves. This condition is open to interpretation, and the person who suffers from it often doesn't agree that they need a guardian. In this case, it's necessary to put together a medical report stating that necessity. Each state has its own laws regarding guardianship/conservatorship, which you need to research before making a decision.

Guardianship—also referred to as conservatorship to differentiate it from cases that involve minor children—can relate to finances and healthcare. Both responsibilities may be designated to the same person or split between two different guardians/conservators. In cases when nobody in the family is available or willing to play that role, the court may appoint someone from outside, always prioritizing the interests of the patient with dementia.

A conservatorship can be established when a family member, friend, or public official asks the court to appoint someone to take care of a person who is unable to handle their finances or make decisions about their personal care. The court will review the request and assign an investigator to assess if the person is truly unable to manage their affairs. The investigator will report back to the court with their findings. The person who needs assistance will have to attend a court hearing unless they are unable to do so due to medical reasons. The judge will then decide if a conservatorship is necessary and what powers the conservator should have. The investigator will continue to check on the person regularly to see if the conservatorship is still needed.

Guardianship/conservatorship processes can be lengthy, involving background checks to make sure that the guardian is fit for the task. A family member often initiates them, then the court assigns an investigator to ensure that the person really is unable to look after themselves. After a hearing in which the patient's presence is necessary—unless they can't attend for medical reasons—the judge decides if guardianship/conservatorship is necessary and what the guardian's powers will be.

By that point, the costs of the process will already be substantial, including the attorney's fees as well as expenses related to legal fees, court filing, and investigator fees—not to mention you now must pay for the guardian's services. The guardian may not be necessary when the patient already has a strong Power of Attorney detailing their wishes. Also, keep in mind that your loved one's details will be in the public record, where anyone can access them.

Despite being costly and time-consuming, guardianship can be worth it. The guardian is a defender of the interests of the person they're looking after. They work as a third party when, for example, the family can't agree on how to manage the patient's assets. They also offer necessary support even when the patient doesn't accept it.

The guardian should be trustworthy, which is why the court will investigate their past for criminal convictions and analyze their credit history. In case no one in the family fulfills that role, or there's a conflict of interest, a public guardian may fit the role. These are usually paid, unlike the family or friend guardians, and need to provide detailed reports of their activities.

An application for guardianship involves the following steps:

1. File an application with the court presenting the required paperwork as provided by the attorney.
2. Inform your family, and anyone who has interest in the loved one, for which you filed the application.
3. Get a doctor to examine the patient and write a report stating that they can't look after themselves and need the assistance of a guardian.
4. Guardian Ad Litem is a legal appointment to determine if a person is incapacitated and needs someone to look after them. It will also determine if the person who's been selected is right for the job.
5. Once the guardian is picked, they accept their job of taking care of the patient with dementia's health and finances.

In case more than one person applies for the role of guardian, the judge may choose one of them or designate each candidate to a different type of guardianship. This will be decided according to the candidate's background and capabilities.

The patient needs a degree of mental competency to create and execute a Power of Attorney. A medical report can confirm that competency, but they can also create a combined mental health declaration and power of attorney stating that all conditions are met. Getting a power of attorney should be one of the first steps you take after the diagnosis. Get an attorney specializing in elderly law to guide you.

Once your loved one is deeper in the dementia process, it becomes harder to get a power of attorney. By then, they might not be able to understand the document and its implications, and you'll have to get help through your local courts to designate the guardian. Through this legal process, you can get the authority to make decisions on their behalf, but it's often expensive and time-consuming. The court may choose a family member, even if they may not necessarily be the most suitable person for the role.

You can also get a durable power of attorney, also known as a financial power of attorney or general power of attorney. Here, a person—usually the spouse or adult child—is appointed to make all decisions on behalf of the person with dementia. This document goes into effect once it's signed and is terminated at the moment of the patient's death. Another option is the medical power of attorney, which deals with decisions related to the patient's health. The medical power of attorney has the power to make decisions regarding the patient's health and what kind of treatment they accept.

Like guardianship, durable power of attorney is directed to the patient's properties and finances or their health and welfare.

These two groups can be designated to two people or a single one. Without a power of attorney, third parties will have to decide on the patient's behalf in an emergency situation. With financial decisions, you might have to take matters into court to be able to, for example, manage your loved one's bank account, modify a loan, or terminate a website subscription. This generates a lot of wasted time that could be avoided with the creation of the power of attorney during the early stages of dementia.

You need to be honest and direct when having a conversation about a power of attorney with your loved one and family members. You can get a durable power of attorney for medical and financial issues at first, which only becomes valid when they lose their capacity to make decisions. Include the advance directive or living will conversation, and be as thorough as possible. Make them understand that the Power of Attorney serves their interests and makes the family's life easier.

Include the power of attorney in the family's conversations during meetings. Some states require that the power of attorney be written, witnessed, and notarized, and someone in the family should be entrusted to take care of that. While the person with dementia is still mentally capable, they can change their power of attorney at any point.

TRUSTS

Creating a living trust for your loved ones allows the family to distribute your loved one's assets without the interference of the law. Living trusts become active as soon as they're established, unlike wills, and are managed by a trustee who will distribute assets among the beneficiaries. A living trust is composed of:

- **Grantor:** the person who creates the trust. They are supposed to take care of documents such as trust documents, trust assets, and insurance policies.
- **Trustees:** The people who manage the trust's assets. Grantors often take this role, but a different trustee should be nominated in case the grantor isn't capable—such as in cases of dementia.
- **Beneficiaries:** People or organizations will receive assets from the trust.

Trusts are often created when a person is still alive, but they can also be created through a will. An irrevocable will can't be changed after its creation, while a revokable will can. This is useful when grantors are still alive and able to make financial decisions—they might change or even cancel the trust.

Revocable trusts are a good way of securing one's future care in case of dementia. The patient with dementia can use it to guarantee the type of care they want, such as home care and assisted living. Revocable trusts are also a practical substitute for both power of attorney and a will, allowing the family to act immediately once the grantor is incapacitated or dies.

Assets are transferred to the trust by the grantor. This involves legally changing the name of the proprietors of such assets from the grantor's name into the name of the trust. This way, the trustee can take control of the trust's financial matters without court intervention. The grantor should still retain some assets to themselves, and it's better to consult with the attorney to determine how much to go into the trust.

The trustee needs to carry out the will of the grantor, which means not using the trust assets for personal purposes or mixing those assets with their own. Each beneficiary should be treated equally unless otherwise instructed in the trust agreement. The trustee is also supposed to take care of the trust's records, file tax returns, and communicate with the beneficiaries when necessary. The trust agreement is their guide, and if they don't follow it, they can be removed from the trust and face legal consequences.

The person or entity that receives and enjoys the trust's assets is called the beneficiary. They may get these assets directly, held in trust, or to pay for the grantor's healthcare expenses—if that's the reason why the trust was created. Death beneficiaries are people who only get access to their share once the grantor passes away. Grantors may be able to use the assets inside the trust while they're still alive if that's specified in the trust agreement. There's a lot of room for misunderstandings, and the terms of the trust must be clear for all participants to avoid conflict.

INTERACTIVE ELEMENT

Hasson (2023) offers the following list of documents that you need to have in hand to solve most legal matters. Mark the ones you have and look for the ones that are missing.

- birth certificate
- marriage certificate
- divorce decree
- citizenship papers
- death certificate of a spouse or parent
- power(s) of attorney
- deeds to property
- deeds to cemetery plots
- military discharge papers
- insurance policies
- pension benefits

It also helps to specify the role of each member of the family in a written document. Write down who will be the designated caregiver, who will oversee, and who will look for additional aid and assistance. Make physical copies of all documents, also keep digital copies stored. All members of the family should know how to access the information.

SEGUE

If you're not a lawyer, legal terms can sound intimidating. It's tempting to get a good attorney and let them deal with all these matters. However, knowing the meaning of those terms and how they can affect your life will prevent you from making blind decisions. Not knowing the law could get you on the wrong track, putting your trust in the wrong place.

The goal of this chapter was to teach you the basics of how the law works. It doesn't replace the services of a good lawyer, but it will help you distinguish one. Now that you have some knowledge of these terms, you won't feel lost when talking to your attorney and will be able to contribute effectively.

With the legal scaffolding now in place, you are better prepared to shield your loved one's assets and ensure their aid eligibility. In the next chapter, we go into how you can use technology to improve your life as a caregiver.

5

TECHNOLOGY AS A CAREGIVER'S ALLY

Technology is best when it brings people together. –Matt Mullenweg

a caregiver living in today's world has at hand a plethora of resources that people didn't dream of a couple of decades ago. This technological revolution has offered digital tools to enhance safety, communication, and quality of life for your loved ones. You can monitor your loved one from short and long distances, get assistance from people around the world, and get exam results in a fraction of the time you'd get them in the past.

People today are more familiar with technology than ever, but the possibilities are still limited. By reading this chapter, you will get to know different resources and be able to select, set up, and utilize a range of technological aids—these range from basic gadgets to advanced equipment, making daily caregiving more manageable and effective. You might have to learn new things, re-learn others that you have already mastered, and adapt them to the needs of your loved one. That's what this chapter is about.

INTRODUCTION TO CAREGIVER TECHNOLOGY

While not everyone can afford to turn their home into a dementia care center, there are more technological solutions available today than ever before. With the democratization of technology, people have turned to their mobile phone apps to look for help regarding their health—both physical and mental. They look for options to alleviate their burden, offer independence to their loved ones, and avoid putting them in a care home. These solutions can help you to support your loved one with dementia if you know how to use them.

You can now find dementia-friendly cell phones and watches that make things easier for your loved one. They are more resistant to damage, offer options such as tracking heart health, and are helpful if your loved one wanders away. You can also assist your loved one with the aid of a plethora of smartphone apps. A quick trip to the Google Play Store or Apple's App Store can give you an idea of what's available. They can help you organize your time, find services, and offer cognitive impairment tests and games to stimulate your mind during moments of distress.

With so many available apps, it's normal to feel overwhelmed or even confused about which ones to use. You may find your phone crowded with dozens of options, while the one that would actually help you remains undiscovered. Some apps may not have been designed for your situation, but they are helpful nonetheless.

Apps such as AmuseIT, Cognitive Therapy, and Lumosity offer games, puzzles, quiz questions, and other pieces of cognitive training that will exercise the patient's memory, logic, and problem-solving skills. They are helpful not only to the dementia patient but also to the caregiver, who can use them to deal with stress and burnout.

A creation of Alzheimer's Research UK, the app A Walk Through Dementia offers a clear idea of what it's like to live with the disease, from doing your daily chores to making important decisions. The Alzheimer's Daily Companion is another Google Play app that offers an important source of training material for caregivers.

Designed specifically for patients with dementia, Mindmate offers valuable information to the caregiver, from games to exercise programs. Another specific program is Iridis, which gives you advice on how to organize your home environment to make it dementia-friendly. A more specific app is Nymbl, which is designed to offer balance training tools to people with dementia to minimize the risk of falling. Its interface is based on 35 years of clinical research, and you need to apply to get access to it.

Other useful apps include:

- It's Done!: An interface that reminds patients of their daily tasks, such as taking their pills or locking a door. Phone or email for more information about the app.
- MyReef 3D Aquarium: A digital aquarium in which the patient can watch and customize a fish tank.
- SingFit: Offers music therapy.

Researchers are currently developing home care robots to assist caregivers. Their goal isn't to replace humans but to offer them assistance, doing housework and playing similar roles to the apps that we've just discussed. These may not be available for a while, and they won't look much like robots in science-fiction movies, but they will become a reality before we know it.

UTILIZING TECHNOLOGY

Assistive technology is a term that encompasses electronic devices used to help memory. They can help you to do your daily tasks and be more independent. While some of them are user-friendly and intuitive, others require some training that you might even get from family or friends who are already familiar with them. These include devices such as Amazon Echo, Google Home, and Apple HomePod, which are voice-activated. They can be used for a plethora of functions, including checking the time and date and reminding that it's medication hour.

You can take advantage of a regular smartphone to program times and dates to alert and remind you of important events. These include reminders that can be customized with different sounds to remind you of a doctor's appointment, that your loved one's favorite TV show is on, or—once again!—of medication time. You can add a text or voice recording to these alarms to remind what they refer to or use a picture taken from your smartphone's camera—the same can be done with a tablet device such as an iPad or Galaxy.

If you are still unsure about giving medication at the right time, you can get a smart medicine dispenser. Once you program them through a smartphone app, they will dispense your loved one's medication at the right time. They also offer reports in case there's a missing dose, which you can monitor remotely.

Getting your loved one an Apple Watch, Google Pixel Watch, or other wearable devices can make it easier for you to track them through GPS. This is helpful if they tend to wander and get lost in crowds. GPS works through a signal that goes from a transmitter to a network of telecommunications satellites. GPS devices are supposed to find anyone anywhere or as far as the satellite signal reaches. Through GPS, you can track where your loved one has been during the day.

Different companies offer different price ranges for their GPS tracker. There are pocket and keychain trackers, which are small and easy to attach to your loved one, as well as wearable trackers, which can be a wrist or ankle band. Be sure that the battery is charged so that you will be able to monitor your loved ones wherever they go.

The GPS tracker will give you peace of mind if, for example, your loved one insists on going to the store on their own. You can monitor their path without having to follow them, making them feel more independent without sacrificing safety. It will also help caregivers have a more active life, being able to track their loved ones while going to the gym or dining out. And if your loved one forgets how to walk back home, you can find them using the coordinates offered by the tracker.

The best GPS options for dementia caregivers include the ability to activate emergency services for your loved one and detect if they wander in an unfamiliar place or if they have fallen, among others. Here are some of the most popular brands:

- Jiobit GPS Tracker
- PocketFinder
- iTraq Nano
- AngelSense GPS Tracker
- Optimus 3.0 GPS Tracker
- TheoraCare GPS Watch
- Geozilla GPS Tracker
- Medical Guardian Freedom GPS Smartwatch
- LandAirSea 54 GPS Tracker
- Trackimo GPS Tracker
- Family1st Elderly GPS Tracker

VIDEO CALLING

Not that long ago, video calling belonged to the realm of science fiction. Now, we have the ability to video chat with people anywhere in the world with excellent quality and no additional costs.

Treating video calling as just a telephone with images would be too simplistic. When you're away from your loved one, a video call could help them remember you and engage in activities that will stimulate their brain. A call software such as Zoom gives you a chance to share your screen, through which you can stream videos, play games, watch a movie together, add more people to the call, and you may end up with a party!

If there is someone who wants to make a video call to your loved one with dementia, it's better to have a pre-session with them. This way, you can give the caller an update about your loved one's condition, including any triggers they shouldn't mention. The person who's calling should know about your loved one's situation, their favorite and least favorite things, and have a good panorama of that person's life to conduct a good conversation.

Always stay by your loved one's side when they're having a video call, no matter how much you trust the person on the screen. Unforeseen things can happen during calls. A weak internet signal can cause distortions and pauses in the video, which can cause distress to your loved one. Something may also happen on the other side of the call.

You can also use video calls to make contact with a health professional. Telehealth makes use of this tool to promote care and support patients without them having to leave home. With the aid of their computer, tablet, or phone, people with mobility impairment can consult with their doctor remotely. It also ensures that caregivers can have access to self-care and education. Telehealth also involves the use of wearable devices to examine a patient. These inform the doctor of the patient's signals and help them monitor mobility and balance issues.

Dementia patients often must consult with specialists, not only in geriatric medicine but in other areas of healthcare. Finding a specialist isn't always easy, and it might require the patient and the caregiver to travel for several hours to meet the doctor. For patients who live in rural areas or who need to commute for hours to see a specialist, Telehealth is a game-changer. It doesn't replace an in-person consultation, in which the doctor can check the vital signs themselves, and any patient should get such a consultation at least once a year. Still, Telehealth is a reality and can offer dignity to people who have a hard time moving around and allow a more thorough examination.

Telehealth proved to be a powerful tool during the COVID-19 pandemic when people had to practice social distancing. It became a popular solution when people were uncomfortable leaving their homes due to the coronavirus. Caregivers couldn't risk taking their loved ones with dementia to hospitals since they were elderly and more vulnerable to the disease. They still needed to consult with doctors and get their treatment, making Telehealth the best solution.

Even after the pandemic, Telehealth has become a good solution for those who, for some reason, can't or won't leave home for simple health concerns such as:

- sinus issues
- urinary problems
- acne, skin rash, or skin infections
- ear pain or discharge
- sore throat and cough
- flu symptoms

- diarrhea, nausea, or vomiting
- questions regarding medication

Even dementia patients who aren't movement-impaired often prefer to stay at home, making Telehealth useful even in post-pandemic times. It makes a difference for them to be examined in the safe and familiar environment of their homes, and medical specialists aren't always keen to physically commute to the patient's house.

To prepare for your appointment, find a spot with good lighting and keep the camera steady. Make sure that the doctor can see your face close to the screen and look straight into the camera. Find a quiet place without background noises, turn off alarms and sounds on other devices, and close other applications on your device. Make the call from a place where you can comfortably discuss your healthcare issues in privacy.

You may take notes on your computer or phone, but good old pen and paper is more reliable and won't distract you from the image on the screen. Use them to write any questions that you may have for your doctor, leaving a space to write their answers. This will give the conversation a clear direction, and you'll be able to get the information you need. Keep notes about the medication being taken, including dosages and the time you take them, so you can pass that information to the doctor without having to rely on your memory. If you can keep the medication with you during the consultation, even better.

Some people will adapt better to Telehealth than others, and that goes for both sides. Remember that an appointment with a doctor isn't a school exam—you can ask them to repeat things as many times as you need to understand. If they go too fast or too slow, you can make a sign that you're going to interrupt them. This is one situation in which you'll be thankful to have a good internet signal. Both sides need to avoid talking on top of the other—that can be awkward in a normal consultation and become chaotic in Telehealth.

When you have to show the doctor pictures, for example, of the patient's body or a health device you use, always take high-resolution photos. They are slower to upload and send, but you want the doctor to have the best image possible. If you still have questions after the appointment, contact the doctor's office. Schedule follow-up care according to the doctor's recommendations. That includes doing lab exams and following their prescription to the letter. Don't hesitate to offer feedback to the provider, whether about the quality of their work or the call, so that they can improve their work.

The doctor is probably busy, and you should show up at the time they have saved for you. You can set your phone to remind you of the time of the appointment, as well as the program you'll use. In some cases, they will lose track of time due to the previous appointment going for longer than they expected. Even then, you should be there on time with all the test results and any materials that the doctor may have requested.

Some insurance providers, such as Medicare, Medicaid, and some private insurance, include Telehealth in their coverage. Coverages vary a lot between states, so research is essential. The quality of the consultation will depend on the quality of your internet signal and devices. Take that into consideration before choosing Telehealth and, if necessary—and affordable—upgrade your technology.

The cost of a Telehealth appointment will vary depending on your insurance status and coverage. Telehealth appointments are covered by Medicare, while private insurance coverage often doesn't differentiate between Telehealth and in-person visits. Call your provider and ask them as many questions as you need. Take into consideration that you will be saving costs that you would have to commute to a doctor's office.

ADAM'S STORY

Nothing that Adam had ever felt in his life compared to the despair of the day his father, George, wandered away. This was the second month after they got the dementia diagnosis, and Adam wasn't sure of what to expect. He knew it was a serious condition, but at the same time, his father had always been a very active man, and it didn't feel right to restrain his freedom.

That afternoon, George said he was going to the bakery. It was only a walk of three blocks, one that he had done often in the past. Adam was busy and didn't notice that George was taking a little longer that day. Then, Adam started to get worried, and he decided to call the bakery. No, he hadn't been there.

Adam made a few more calls before deciding to get in his car and look for his dad around the neighborhood. It took him twenty minutes, and he found George sitting on a bench, staring at the ground. No harm had been done that time, but Adam promised he would be more careful.

His first thought was not to let George go out alone at all. If George wanted to go to the bakery, Adam would either go with him or tell him not to go. That wasn't going to work for long, so Adam decided to do some research and found the solution in a GPS tracker, which he attached to George's keychain. Now that he knew where his dad was at any time of the day, things became much easier without sacrificing anyone's freedom.

Here's a list of technological devices that you can use to make your life as a caregiver easier. Check the ones you're already using, and consider acquiring some of the others.

- adaptive clocks
- adaptive telephones
- adaptive clothing
- appliance use monitors
- augmented reality glasses
- automated pill dispensers
- dementia-friendly speakers
- eating aids
- electric razors
- elevated toilets
- in-home video monitors
- location trackers
- medical alerts devices
- robotic pets
- simple phones or tablets aid in two-way talks
- sliding transfer seat
- smart home devices help with supervision
- telepresent robots
- three-sided toothbrush
- voice reminders
- wearable detection devices

Here are some smartphone apps for patients with dementia. Check the ones you've already used.

- Carezone
- Iridis
- It's Done!

- Let's Create! Pottery
- Mindmate
- My Reef 3D Aquarium

SEGUE

The most useful scientific discoveries are translated into technology that can make our lives happier, healthier, and more efficient. They also serve to make already-existing inventions more user-friendly, opening doors for new experiences. In the modern world, it's easy to become so dependent on technology that we can't remember how things used to be before we had access to it.

We dedicated this chapter to exploring technological options that can improve your life as a caregiver. You learned how to make the best out of simple devices and how to use more advanced ones. We also explored the world of smartphone apps and how you can find one to fulfill almost any need.

With the digital world now at your fingertips, it's time to turn to your living space. In the next chapter, we'll take the principles of tech-savvy care to the next level, ensuring every corner of your home supports the well-being of your loved one with dementia.

6

CREATING A SMART AND SAFE HOME ENVIRONMENT

A house is made of walls and beams; a home is built with love and dreams. –Ralph Waldo Emerson

*M*ost seniors want to stay in their homes as they age–how does smart technology make that wish a reality? You never know how disaster-prone your home can be until you have to deal with little children, pets, or elderly people. The latter case is worse if the person is suffering from dementia and has trouble recognizing everyday items such as a knife, a telephone cord, or an electrical socket, all of which can end up in disaster.

Once you decide where your loved one is going to live, it's time to start adapting the house to their needs. Transforming a living space into a dementia-friendly environment is easier with the help of smart technology, but it takes work and determination. In this chapter, you'll find out how to choose and implement smart devices that offer enhanced safety and comfort for dementia patients, ultimately fostering a sense of autonomy and well-being.

THE APPEAL OF STAYING AT HOME

Sauer (2018) mentions an AARP study according to which 90% of the senior population don't want to move from their homes for the next decade. Of those, 85% are aware that they need to make changes to their home since they have trouble living by themselves. According to this research, only 43% assume they can live by themselves without much trouble.

The reasons for wanting to stay at home vary from person to person, but the stress of moving to a new place is a decisive factor. This process can be distressing for anyone, and it can also involve looking for a new place and possibly losing precious belongings during the move. It's not just about losing objects, but about saying goodbye to their home.

Moving away also means saying goodbye to a community and being open to meeting new people, shopping in new stores, learning new routes, and reconfiguring one's entire routine. There's a reason why children hate moving to a new neighborhood, and it's the same for the elderly, except that they can be even more fragile.

At times, elderly people must leave their own homes to move in with their children, which can rob everyone of their sense of independence. The same happens when they're moved into a care facility, where nurses and other staff members monitor everything they do. Staying in their own house means keeping that independence and sense of empowerment.

At a certain age, people generally become averse to change. For some elderly people, including patients with dementia, fighting that fight inside a place they know is less scary than doing it in strange territory. However, there are many situations in which *not* moving away isn't an option. Maybe the costs of keeping the home are prohibitive, or they find the patient with dementia may need intensive care they maybe cannot get when living at home.

It can be hard to convince your loved one that they need to move into a care home. They may not accept it, even if you argue that it will cut costs for the family and that they will get everything they need from a trained staff. They will also be surrounded by people of their age and can get visits from family and volunteers who are there to engage with the patients.

In some situations, the patient with dementia will have to leave their home to stay with members of the family. This move can be stressful for all parties, even if everyone has good relations. As loving and caring as the family may be, people with dementia can be a real challenge, especially as the disease progresses, and it can be devastating to see this decline happening in front of your eyes. Children will notice there's something wrong with their grandparents, and at this point, if they are old enough to understand, open up to them and explain what's happening instead of pretending everything is alright.

Try to see things through their eyes. If the place they lived is well known to you, try to think of how they would adapt to the new situation. If they're moving to your house, take a walk around the place and try to see things from their point of view. How would they interact with the stairs, the bathroom, the carpet, the curtains? Is there any noise, smell, or visual element that could cause them discomfort? What would be the most difficult things for them to adapt, and what changes are you ready to make to minimize their discomfort.

Some changes are as small as moving pieces of furniture around or removing a rug. Others are more dramatic and can affect the rest of the family. Getting help from geriatric experts and doctors will help you make better decisions. Keep in mind that as your loved one's condition progresses, you may have to make more changes. Keep a notebook to write down observations about which changes worked and which didn't. Use that to plan for future ones.

You can't monitor your loved one at every moment of night and day, but you can make sure that the environment is safe. While it's not ideal that they wander around the house by themselves, you should make sure they can get in and out of bed without effort, avoiding potential falls and injury. They should have a bell or a horn by the bed to call for your assistance, and you can use a baby monitor to check if everything is okay in the bedroom. Motion-activated lights are also useful to avoid injuries as they look for the light switch on the wall.

The bathroom is one of the most dangerous places in a common household for people with dementia. There are special appliances designed to keep them safe. Bathing seats can be installed in showers and bathtubs to make bathing time more practical. You also want to install grab bars in that area to help patients with dementia sit down and stand up.

Automatic faucets activated by motion guarantee that you won't let water run by accident, which could cause slippery floors. Some faucets also come with temperature control to avoid scalding, which is a serious problem with elderly people. There are nonskid bath mats that minimize the chance of slipping, which you can install all around the house, but especially in the bathroom. Finally, remove the locks from the bathroom doors. Even if you've installed all these safety items, you don't want them to lock themselves in there.

The bathroom might be the most accident-prone area of the house, but the kitchen offers just as many dangers. Always keep an eye on the food you're serving your loved one, for their bodies may be more vulnerable to spoiled food. Everyday items such as garbage disposals, blenders, mixers, food processors, coffee makers, air fryers, toasters, and microwaves could cause accidents, and it's better to disconnect them when they're not being used. Just as dangerous are the knives, forks, skewers, and other appliances that could cut or bruise your loved one. Keep them stored securely when you're not using them.

The main danger in the kitchen is burns, and they can happen even if your loved one doesn't have direct access to the stove. Be careful when serving them food on hot plates, and if possible, keep them away from the kitchen while you're dealing with fire or hot water.

Accidents may happen in the living room as well, so it's best to always have your shelves and bookcases attached to the walls. That will prevent them from falling over if your loved one bumps into furniture. If you're not an organized person, this is the time to start. Keeping each item in your living room in the right place is an important step to ensure safety. Also, don't leave electric outlets exposed, but instead, cover them with child-proof plastic plug covers to avoid electric shocks.

A house with a backyard is great to provide your loved one with some recreation, as long as you adapt it first. Remove anything where they can slip on or stumble into, such as stones, hose, moss, and puddles of rain. The area should be well-lit during night and day, if possible, with motion-activated spotlights, and you can install rubber mats to make the pavement safer. It's also important that the backyard has fences with latches to prevent your loved one from wandering off the premises.

Glass doors are a danger to run into. At best, your loved one will bruise their heads, and at worst, they will break the door and cut themselves. This can be solved by marking the glass door with bright tape at their eye level. In case your house has large wall mirrors, you might consider removing them. The illusion caused by the reflection could create cognitive confusion in the patient with dementia, leading to anxiety and panic attacks.

ADAPTING TO NEEDS

A dementia patient needs a safe, comfortable, and familiar environment that promotes independence and reduces confusion and distress. This will help them fulfill their daily activities with less distress and reduce the chance of an accident.

Improving the lighting throughout the home is a good place to start. Without adequate lighting, you risk creating confusion and the risk of falls. This is not just about getting more light in strategic places—though that's crucial—but also installing automatic light sensors activated by motion. They are helpful if your loved one decides to walk around the house in the middle of the night and may get confused trying to find the light switch. Making your floor a matte color that contrasts with your walls will help patients with dementia differentiate between them as they move around the house.

Adapting your home to a patient with dementia can be as simple as buying a phone with large buttons. But you can also go the extra mile and turn your house into a smart house. That means getting a series of devices that make your life easier, such as remote locking systems, voice-activated appliances, and smart thermostats that keep your house at the right temperature, whether or not you are at home.

A cluttered home can be like a minefield for a person with dementia. Most of us are used to zigzag around certain objects and furniture in our house. Some of them have their utility, but a lot of them are just there to take up space. Decluttering the house means creating a safer environment.

The house must be well-lit with both natural and artificial light. Not only because it allows people to know where they're going but also to see, recognize, and interpret facial expressions and understand body language. This helps your loved one to remember who their loved ones much longer.

Sunlight aids the production of Vitamin D, which influences mood and sleep. Still, you don't want too much light entering the house, making it too hot and causing glares and reflections that can disorient your loved one. You can control how much light enters your window with a good set of blinds and curtains.

Keep important objects at hand in visible places so your loved one can find them whenever they need them. If they want a glass of water—preferably one made of plastic—they should be able to find the right glass. You could get a cabinet with a see-through door and, if that's not possible, label each door with a drawing of what your loved one will find inside it. You can also install clocks around the house, making sure they are synchronized. Knowing what time it is reduces anxiety and makes people feel more in control.

SMART HOME

The concept of a smart home involves controlling many things via Wi-Fi from a mobile app. These are usually easy to install, coming with a specific app that you can download on your phone. Some will require a more complex installation, with low-voltage wiring and drilling—in which case you might want to hire a professional installer. Some of them are voice-activated.

Improving your home for your loved one isn't just about changing the physical structure of the house and installing safety devices. It can also be about getting everything connected so you can give them the best possible assistance from anywhere. This isn't always cheap, and you might need to get the help of a professional. You don't have to buy a whole new set of home appliances to have a smart home. You can optimize ordinary serves through a smart plug, allowing you to control lamps, lights, TVs, and other items through your phone.

Smart devices designed to assist patients with dementia are available in stores or online. They are created to prevent accidents and to make the lives of the patient and their caregiver easier and more practical. Artificial intelligence is available in some systems. These can learn the typical routine of the house, identifying, for example, deviations in sleeping patterns or irregular meal times.

It might take some time for you and your loved one to get used to a smart home. Introducing these changes gradually will avoid confusion or distress. At first, it will feel like your life is being watched and controlled by these devices, but with time, you will learn to rely on them. Smart homes serve to adapt your living environment to your habits. A self-adjusting thermostat, for example, learns which temperature you prefer and adjusts itself accordingly.

Caregivers can rely on this technology to support them in many situations, while patients with dementia can rely on it to keep some of their independence. While the disease affects the abilities of learning, perception, memory, and problem-solving, a smart house addresses these challenges and offers new options. Most of us are used to light bulbs that can be turned on or off. With smart bulbs, you can control color, temperature, and brightness levels from your phone to create different ambiances for different occasions.

Voice control is one of the most dynamic features of a smart house. With a voice command, you can turn the lights on or off, adjust the air conditioning, change the volume of the radio, make a cup of tea, and much more. Smart speakers give access to popular voice assistants such as Amazon Alexa, Apple Siri, and Google Assistant.

The home environment is different from that of a lab or a factory, which is where these devices were first used. In a factory, each robot performs a programmed task that can be easily quantified. A home has many variables, such as the position of the furniture, the different people who interact with it, and the unpredictable nature of dementia itself. Because of that, a smart home isn't supposed to do everything for everyone but to teach how they act in the environment and give support when needed.

You can manage your air conditioning and heating via your phone with smart thermostats. They adapt the temperature according to the time of the day, your whereabouts, and the status of other connected devices through remote room sensors. Installation is generally straightforward, involving low-voltage wiring and minimal drilling.

Smart locks allow you to lock and unlock your door using your phone, and many offer the ability to manage access for different individuals, including friends, family, and workers. Some smart locks even support voice commands for locking and unlocking doors, while others provide fingerprint access. Most smart locks come as complete sets that are easy to install, although a few models only require replacing a single interior component.

Smart technology is also a game changer concerning security. With a smart doorbell, you can see and communicate with visitors on your front step before deciding whether to open the door. Powered models that can be installed in minutes without any wiring. Smart cameras use motorized components that allow them to have a 360-degree view, moving according to sensors. Their footage can be recorded locally or saved online.

You can integrate that audio and video into your phone and record it. It's also possible to connect your phone to motion detection sensors and alarms. Battery cameras require minimal installation work and little to no drilling.

To make your smart home work, a reliable Wi-Fi connection is essential. Wi-Fi is becoming more secure, using less power, and handling more devices. All of this makes it more suitable for a smart home where you don't want congestion of Wi-Fi signals interfering with each other. It's wise to keep the smart home devices in a separate network and create a strong password for it.

You can control some smart home devices through Bluetooth or a special smart hub, such as Philips Hue bulbs. While these methods aren't as fast and reliable as Wi-Fi, their signals are less crowded and less prone to congestion. You can have them as a second and third option for your devices in case you lose your Wi-Fi signal.

ENGAGING ACTIVITIES

Technology is an ally, but the human factor will always play the lead role in dealing with a patient with dementia. Their environment must be comforting, but it must also stimulate them to connect with those around them. With simple daily activities, it's possible to make them feel more at home as dementia progresses and they struggle with learning new things.

All people can benefit from the sense of control that a strict routine provides. It keeps you active even when you don't feel like doing much, provides you with focus, and gets you ready for new experiences. It also gives a structure to the day, which offers a sense of direction and stability, thus reducing stress and anxiety.

You can apply all of that to your loved one by establishing their daily activities. Implementing that routine at the beginning of the disease will give you better results. This goes beyond having time to brush their teeth or go to bed—you should include art projects, games, outdoor exercises, music, and other activities that they can follow and recognize with pleasure.

Lundberg (2023) offers the following list of activities that can be used with a patient with dementia:

- experiment with sounds
- encourage visual expression
- explore sensory craft experiences
- create collages
- relive the past with classic movies and TV shows
- listen to music and sing
- look through photo albums
- journey back in time
- fold laundry
- engage in handy activities
- untie knots
- do a puzzle
- play a game
- stop and smell the roses
- touch the past
- feel diverse textures
- discover nature and art through live cams
- venture globally with Google Earth
- create a family video tablet for dementia patients at home

Not every patient will react well to all of these activities. Be watchful as you implement them, and identify when they look happy and engaged or distracted, anxious, or irritated. It can be frustrating to realize that the activity you planned so carefully doesn't please your loved one, but if that's the case, it is best to switch to something else.

Timing each activity to the right time of the day is crucial to its success. Your loved one may enjoy watching old movies on TV, but you shouldn't let them have much screen time right before going to bed. This time is more suitable for listening to calm music or feeling textures.

Offer as much physical and mental activity as your loved one can handle without getting overwhelmed. Choose activities that suit the abilities your loved one already has. Learning new things can be difficult and frustrating, even if you're young and you don't want to expose your loved one to that. Don't criticize or correct them if they don't do something right—this isn't about being perfect!

INTERACTIVE ELEMENT

Here's a safe home checklist to help you identify items that may include technology.

- motion-activated lights
- motion-activated alarms
- use a pool cover
- cover electric outlets
- automatic faucets
- grab bars
- remove locks from bathroom doors
- nonskid bath mats
- clocks around the house
- baby monitor
- adaptive furniture
- reliable Wi-Fi
- Bluetooth

In this chapter, we've learned that our loved ones prefer to stay in their own familiar homes. However, as familiar as that place might be, it can offer many dangers that could harm your loved one. Being aware of those dangers is the first step in preventing accidents from happening.

Just as your loved one's mind is changing, their home also needs to change to adapt to their new needs. By using the right equipment, you can offer them the best experience and make your own life a lot easier. We now have access to technology that goes beyond what science fiction had predicted. Still, it's vital to remember that technology is only as powerful as the comfort it brings. They haven't yet invented a machine that can offer love and understanding to another human being.

In the next chapter, we'll explore how to balance the high-tech with the high-touch, ensuring that you, too, receive the support you need to thrive on this caregiving journey.

7

EMOTIONAL AND PRACTICAL
SUPPORT FOR CAREGIVERS

Self-care is not a selfish act—it is good stewardship of the only gift I have, the gift I was put on earth to offer to others. –Parker Palmer

ou are not a machine. There's nothing wrong with questioning your decisions, feeling overwhelmed, and crying from time to time. As a caregiver, you have many responsibilities that are not always easy to meet. You also have to watch the decline of the mental and physical health of your loved one, and that's a huge burden in itself.

Resist the urge to ignore that and put all of your focus on your work. Those feelings will surface, perhaps at a bad time, and you will pay for not taking care of your mental health. Looking for equilibrium in your daily life is part of what makes you a good caregiver and is as important to your loved one as it is to you.

It's necessary to recognize the importance of dementia care as a public health priority, with the aging population on the rise and different forms of dementia posing a burden. The World Health Organization highlights the need for increased support to family caregivers, who often play a central role in providing care. However, caring for someone with dementia can be a long-term and stressful responsibility, which can lead to depression among family caregivers.

In this chapter, you will learn to recognize and address the emotional challenges that accompany the role of caring for a loved one with dementia. Here, you'll learn effective stress management techniques, receive practical advice for self-care, and gain access to a comprehensive directory of support resources. With this, you'll create a support system that sustains your emotional well-being through your caregiving journey.

THE EMOTIONAL TOLL OF CAREGIVING

Depression, or melancholia, is an emotional disorder that comes in many forms. In its mildest form, it can be confused with disappointment caused by loss. As it develops, it can become a serious issue that harms people's personal, social, and professional lives. There are many treatments for depression, though there's still a lot of prejudice against them.

Caregivers are often called invisible second patients, for they suffer the consequences of dementia indirectly. They also need a certain amount of care, which is not often acknowledged by those around them, who are more concerned about the person who has an actual medical diagnosis. Caregivers are subject to emotional breakdown and the health problems that follow a low immune system caused by stress. Yet, people tend to overlook that until the last minute.

Different forms of dementia are developing as the elderly population continues to grow. It's important that the family plays an important role at this stage of their life. It isn't an easy task, and most people aren't prepared for the long term.

Family caregivers choose to provide care for their loved ones for different reasons. For some, it's a noble mission guided by a sense of giving back or duty. In most cases, they like and get along with the person who they're taking care of. In others, they don't, but they learn to as they battle together against this disease. Others do it out of a sense of guilt or familial pressure. Caregiving isn't necessarily a negative experience and can lead to spiritual and personal growth. For those who can't afford to pay for professional help, caring for a loved one with dementia can bring a sense of purpose and the satisfaction of a job well done.

Caregiving is a full-time job that requires different functions. This includes the ones the caregiver must do by themselves and the ones they can or must coordinate with other professionals, such as a visiting nurse, doctors, physical therapists, and others. As time goes by, these necessities change, and it is the job of the caregiver to identify new necessities and find the best way of addressing them.

Distributing tasks isn't uncommon in most households. However, one person is often designated as the main caregiver, with most day-to-day activities delegated to them. The other members of the family are allowed to go on with their careers and social life and will hopefully be there in the harshest moments and offer financial support to their loved ones.

The psychological burden can lead caregivers to sacrifice their personal projects, interests, and hobbies. Whether it's a professional career, a book they want to read, an instrument they'd like to play, or a simple walk in the park on the weekends—they may have little to no energy to do any of that. It's important that their family and friends encourage them to do what makes them happy.

Several issues can influence how stressful the caregiving experience will be. Information is a key factor since people who (unlike you!) don't educate themselves about dementia will have to learn as they go along—which can be exhausting. Stress is also common in people who don't have a solid network to help them.

Not everyone is ready to face dementia when it first appears. Some will deny it to themselves or others. In some cases, because they want to believe their loved one is alright, in others because they don't have enough confidence in that person, think they are just making a play for attention. That leads to frustration and anger and will have an impact on the patient with dementia.

As the reality of dementia settles, caregivers may want to stay away from social affairs. They may not want to explain to their friends what's going on and may prefer to have time for themselves and for the person they're caring for. However, being alone increases the anxiety of what's to come and makes them question if they're doing enough. That's when depression hits hard.

There's nothing more frustrating than the feeling of not being able to complete small daily tasks. When depression goes untreated, personal tasks are the first to suffer, such as housecleaning and the dishes. How can one do anything with a mind full of concerns? There's still a sick person who needs to be taken care of, though. With so many things that can happen during the night, getting a good night's sleep can be difficult.

By this point, the caregiver can't concentrate on much and starts making more mistakes. They can be irritated after many sleepless nights and can't remember the last time they've been relaxed. This will take a toll not only on their mental health but also on their body, making them more susceptible to illness.

When the burden of depression becomes too much, the caregiver might need an intervention from their loved ones. The effects of the intervention aren't always great, but they might be necessary if the person is getting too affected by the situation. The most effective kind of intervention is the psycho-educational one. It involves training about dementia and the best ways of dealing with its effects. This plays an active part in the caregiver's daily life and helps to alleviate their burden.

When preparing an intervention, it's necessary to respect the uniqueness of each caregiver. Some of them prefer individualized therapy, while others work better in intervention groups. When the caregiver is an elderly individual, they may resist talking to a therapist or taking anti-depressants. Anyone may feel this way.

TECHNIQUES FOR STRESS MANAGEMENT AND SELF-CARE

Knowing how to use healthcare and social services makes a difference in the caregiving journey. They serve not only to get access to specialists and medication but also to offer caregiver training and emotional support. Knowing the right coping strategies is important to fight the stress of being a caregiver.

Don't deny yourself the choice of being positive. That feeling may sound unrealistic in this scenario, almost as if you closing your eyes to what's happening to your loved one. Instead, it's about approaching each issue with a can-do attitude, focusing on finding solutions instead of stressing about a problem that seems hopeless.

No matter how stressed you are right now or how many mistakes you have made—it's not too late to turn this into a positive experience! Think of yourself as the most important asset in caring for your loved one. Like any asset, you need care.

There are more options now to cope with stress than ever before, thanks to the internet. You can find web-based courses, research new ways of coping with stress, and have online sessions with therapists if you can't commute to an office.

Some people can recognize that stress is affecting their minds, yet they continue to push themselves past that point. At first, they might feel like a sign of strength, but it takes its toll as the effects become more apparent. Knowing when to stop is important, but as a caregiver, it's not always a choice. Crises will happen when you must put everything aside and dedicate 100% to your loved one. Still, when you start feeling overwhelmed, it's wise to schedule an appointment with your doctor and, ideally, get therapy sessions through your support system. More on that later.

Don't wait until you have a panic attack or start to become aggressive with those around you, as that could affect the treatment of your loved one. There are simple exercises you can do, like screaming in a stack of pillows or breathing exercises. These don't replace regular medical treatment, but they can help you to control your mood during difficult times.

Other things you can try include:

- **Meditation**
- **Massages**
- **Yoga**: You can attend paid yoga courses, but there are also yoga groups that gather in public places such as parks and squares, where you can enjoy these exercises for free.
- **Progressive muscle relaxation**: First, tighten, then relax each muscle group, starting from the feet and working your way to the top of your head.
- **Visualization**: Mentally picturing a place or situation that is peaceful and calm.

- **Physical activity**: Reduces stress and provides a feeling of well-being. It can be as simple as going for a walk.
- **Gardening**: Dealing with plants and getting your hands dirty can be relaxing.
- **Dancing**: Not only does it keep you moving, it also allows artistic expression. You can get dance classes, go out to dance, or just put some music on a speaker at your home and lose yourself!
- **Playing a musical instrument**: You don't have to be good enough to play in a band, but making some music will help you to relax and have time for yourself.

You can also find satisfaction in the time and effort you spend to become a better caregiver, taking courses, reading books, and talking to other people who are in a similar situation. Embracing your current situation will give you a sense of purpose and keep your mind away from feeling helpless. Having a sense of humor can also do wonders—not in the sense of laughing at tragedy, but of looking at things in a lighter way.

Manage your expectations, and always have in mind that you're only human. Nobody can expect you to do more than the best you can—even if, at some moments, that's not enough. Caregivers are often thrown into this situation without preparation, which is hard for anyone. Be nice to yourself, even—and especially!—if others aren't.

At times, you'll feel that you can't solve a huge problem. The best approach is to divide that problem into smaller tasks and tackle them one at a time. You don't need to have everything figured out for a year or even a week from now. Everything could change by then, and you need to do what works for the moment.

Enjoy the quiet times that you spend with your loved one. You can watch television together, look at old photos, and have warm conversations—as long as you respect their loss of memory. Keep in mind that no matter how good a job you do, your loved one will still have health problems caused by the illness. Though you can't prevent that, you can help them through that situation.

Find comfort in the thought that you are making a difference by caring for someone who can't take care of themselves. You may not be a superhero for the world, but you are for that person. At times, you'll wish there was more you could do, but don't force yourself beyond your breaking point.

It's comprehensible that you feel powerless about the situation as the condition progresses. Every caregiver experiences that and the feeling that they are losing their loved one. If you need to cry, go to a place where your loved one can't see or hear you and cry as much as you need. Then dry your face and go back to work.

If your loved one does something that bothers or annoys you, try to put yourself in their shoes. A sense of spirituality can get you through tough situations. Some people find comfort in going to a church, temple, or mosque and attending a religious service. Others prefer to develop their spirituality by them-selves, finding strength in their faith in a higher power.

One of the most powerful allies against stress is consulting mental health professionals. Going to a weekly one-hour appointment and discussing what's bothering you can do wonders for your mental health. Most insurance plans provide mental health coverage. Check your policy to verify your benefits.

STRATEGIES FOR LEVERAGING RESOURCES

There are plenty of resources for those dealing with dementia if you know how to look for them. First, you and your family need to sit with pen and paper in hand and write the things you need help with at the beginning, your doubts about how this will go, and the needs you might have in the future.

With that list in hand, you can start building your support network. You might have someone in the family with good health insurance, which you could extend to their loved one. Your next-door neighbor might be a good home cook who would appreciate some extra money to double their portions and share it. You'd be surprised with how many people are willing to help if only you asked them.

People don't need to be physically near you to offer their help. Family members can communicate through Zoom video calls from anywhere in the world. That granddaughter who moved to another state or even another continent to go to college can still keep in touch with their granny and grandpa through weekly calls.

Take advantage of the community care programs and services created to help people with chronic health conditions, including dementia. They can help with household chores, offer emotional support to you and your loved one, and support a vibrant social and recreational life. This service is provided by people who have a background in social work and healthcare and who will be there for you in crises. You can get your loved one into a community adult daycare program. There, they can receive medical assistance and socialize while alleviating your burden if you can't look after them 24 hours a day.

The quality and availability of all those services may change from one location to another, and it's not always easy to meet the eligibility requirements. It can be tiresome to contact community care and get the services you need, so start while things are still under control. You might be put on a waiting list, which could be a problem in an emergency.

Here are some of the ways technology can help you as a caregiver:

- **Coordinating care:** Have a page or group in an app such as WhatsApp where members of the family can get together and talk about any issues regarding caregiving. You can manage appointments, distribute tasks, organize visits, and keep everyone together.
- **Medication management:** Set up an alarm on your phone with the time and the name of each medication that your loved one is supposed to take.
- **Record tracking:** There are apps in which you can record events related to the health of your loved one. You can register the time each symptom manifested, how long it took for them to fall asleep, how many times they went to the toilet, and other information that can be valuable for doctors.
- **Psychological support:** Caregivers often feel isolated, and online connections can help with that feeling. Not only can you keep in touch with your family and friends through social apps, but you can also enter groups of people who are in a similar situation.
- **Meditation:** When stress reaches high levels, you can take 10-15 minutes alone and use a meditation app. These use sounds of nature, calming music, and mantras that will help you relax.
- **Spirituality:** Caregivers don't always have the chance to commute to a worshipping site and often lose contact with their spirituality. If that's your case, look for an app

that suits you, and take a few minutes a day to get in touch with your spiritual side.

- **Information:** An educated caregiver will do their job with less stress. There are webinars that you can access online, and you can find one for any subject in the world, including how to become a better caregiver.
- **Safety:** We've seen how GPS trackers and other wearables can help to locate your loved one in case they wander out of the house or monitor their health. As a caregiver, you may find that a wearable may be equally beneficial to you.
- **Exercise:** It's hard to find time to take care of your physical health when you have to take care of a patient with dementia. You may promise yourself you'll go for a walk every day but only remember about it by the time you go to bed. Set an alarm for when it's exercising time and enlist someone to stay with your loved one at that specific time.
- **Shopping:** Running errands can become impossible when you are dedicated to taking care of your loved one. Shopping for goods and services online is a good option, from getting groceries to paying bank bills and getting new clothes and other items.
- **Entertainment:** Getting time to watch a movie or a series will help you to organize your mind. You don't have to physically go to a movie theater to see a movie or wait for the right day and hour to watch your favorite series.

Here are some social media site resources you can use:

- **Facebook:** Where you can create a page for your loved one and add family members so they can keep track of what's going on or join groups that are of interest, including caregiver support.

- **X** (previously known as Twitter): Here, you can follow specialists in dementia and get new information about research and other news.
- **Pinterest, Discord, and Yelp:** This helps you to save and pinpoint items and information that you find useful and enjoyable that you need to access again later on.

ELVIN'S STORY

For Elvin Tan, taking care of his mother with dementia and his older brother with schizophrenia had become a life mission. So much so that he isolated himself from family and friends and decided to face this battle alone. As time went by, Elvin's mental health became an issue, with no one he could talk to about his battle.

It came to a point when he couldn't take anymore, and he decided to attend caregiver support and start taking classes on caregiving. Suddenly, Elvin realized he wasn't alone in this journey, that many others were facing the same issues as him, and that this road had been traveled before.

With Elvin's story, we learned that there's no point in trying to do this alone and that looking for help doesn't make your journey less valid.

INTERACTIVE ELEMENT

Here are the main signs that you need to start reaching out for support. Mark the ones that fit your situation:

- getting irritated easily
- not caring for your health

- a constant feeling of worry
- sleeping too much or not enough
- feeling sad and tired all the time
- a dramatic weight change
- excessive numbing using alcohol or drugs
- having frequent pain

If you ticked one or more of these, it's time to look for help through your support group or a professional.

SEGUE

We started this chapter with the words: *You are not a machine.* A machine is designed to fulfill a task endlessly and without assistance. A human being is much more complex, with strengths and weaknesses, and will break if treated like a machine.

Being a caregiver is tough, and you can't afford a mental breakdown, for that will have an effect on your loved one, as well. Self-care is an important part of that process, and in this chapter, we've seen some of the ways you can watch out for your mind, body, and spirit enabling you to become stronger and more resilient and—why not?—happy as you go on with your daily life.

These strategies for emotional resilience and a support system will prepare you for what lies ahead. In the next chapter, we'll look to the future, giving you foresight and planning tools to provide compassionate care as your loved one's journey with dementia evolves.

8

NAVIGATING THE FUTURE
TOGETHER

They may forget what you said, but they will never forget how you made them feel. −Carl Buechner

*L*ooking back, the patterns of our journey become clearer. We understand not only the mistakes we made and the things we could have done better but also the moments in which we accomplished more than we thought possible. This is a journey of pain and frustration, love and tough choices, but also of hope and self-discovery.

It helps to look at your journey as an evolving landscape. You will have to adapt care plans as your loved one's condition progresses. It's important to communicate with healthcare providers about the future, be open to looking at things as they are, and face tough news when necessary. As the condition progresses, you will have to incorporate new medical developments in your care strategies, which means dealing with new professionals and procedures.

Dementia will affect the behavior and personality of your loved one, making them act unlike their old self. People with dementia will also perceive the environment in a different way, causing anger and confusion as the patient can't follow what's going on around them. They can be overstimulated by simple noises and conversations that they cannot process. They are also vulnerable to emotional cues, which can cause anxiety and worry. In some cases, those feelings are caused by medical issues, especially if they can't communicate to others what they're feeling.

Healthcare providers can identify the source of irritation through exams that detect issues such as pain caused by diseases, injuries, or infections. Some of these issues can be treated with medication, but in many cases, you'll have to change your daily routine and way of interacting with your loved one. Calm and patience are the key.

In some cases, problems may be easy to solve, like the bedroom temperature, disorienting lighting, or difficulty finding the bathroom. You need to keep a consistent environment where the person with dementia can find what they need, with a well-lit environment that doesn't project too many shadows and a furniture arrangement that avoids accidents.

Review your arrangements to make sure your loved one isn't going to bed too early or getting too much sleep during the day, all of which could make them tired. You can solve this by engaging them with increased physical activity within their abilities, such as a simple walk, and avoiding giving them too much caffeine or alcohol.

Dementia isn't an integral part of aging. People can reach over a hundred years of age without any signs of dementia. Like with any disease, it isn't an isolated occurrence, and it can be caused or facilitated by other health factors. The risk of dementia can be changed or reduced by taking into account certain factors, such as high blood pressure, smoking, alcohol abuse, depression, obesity, low activity levels, diabetes, and level of social interaction. Dementia also tends to appear in cases of traumatic brain injury and can be caused by breathing polluted air.

Some families try to protect their loved ones from the world around them, they keep them from staying cognitively, physically, and socially active. However, the lack of those interactions, including physical and cognitive exercise, can cause depression and lead to obesity, diabetes, and cardiovascular risk. When you, for example, restrict an elderly person from taking care of their garden as they've done for years and instead have them sit on the couch all day staring at the walls, their minds become more susceptible to advanced dementia.

The goal of dementia care is to guarantee the well-being of the patient. It not only keeps them clean and fed but also makes them enjoy their daily life, feel motivated, and have fun—all of which decrease the level of depression. Treatment needs to be tailored to each patient's needs and symptoms to maintain their physical and mental health. The level of hospitalizations of elderly people with dementia is higher than for people of the same age who don't have it. The distress caused by this process affects their dementia, causing some to develop delirium and get confused about the world around them.

Advance care planning is a complicated process, and you need to change strategies constantly as dementia progresses. It means discussing and keeping records of the wishes and values of the patients. These records can be used later when the patient can no longer speak for themselves. A crucial part of dementia palliative care, advance care planning is a recent concept. It offers the patient the right to know what's going on with them and be part of future decisions when they can no longer make decisions for themselves.

Caregivers are put in a position where they have to make legal and medical decisions about issues they don't fully comprehend —unless they're doctors and lawyers themselves. These decisions will also be influenced by their relationship with the patient. They might not understand how serious dementia is and how fast their loved ones may lose their cognitive abilities.

Like dementia, advanced care planning changes progressively, and the rate changes during the process. You have to document the changes in your loved one's habits and determine when they're not capable of doing something. It may take a while for you to notice, for example, that they can't use a fork by themselves. Once that's established, you can take the proper action.

When the family of a patient with dementia is caught off guard in a situation like this, it's the healthcare provider's job to introduce the concept of advanced care planning to them. Once the doctor and the family are on the same page, they can start working together, keeping regular appointments to discuss the progression of the disease. You will have to take your loved one to many specialists, and having professionals that you can stick to during the entire process will offer you reassurance.

Dementia caregivers tend not to start advance care planning at the right time, either because they don't understand the seriousness of the disease, feel insecure about the subject, or are not properly instructed. Patients often resist starting the process for fear of the future that's implied in the documents.

All of this can be solved with proper education about the effects of dementia and what advanced care planning is all about. Dialogue from all parties involved helps to create an understanding of what's to come and how this is the best way of preparing for that. It's a delicate subject, but it can't be treated as taboo. Your loved one needs to understand that, by recording their wishes and preferences regarding their care, they will be respected.

In this situation, both patients and caregivers need to rework their mindset. The help of a professional is essential, but you can also find knowledge in a person who has gone through the same situation or by reading a book like this one. There are no easy answers, and it's impossible to fully prepare for the road ahead. That doesn't have to be scary or bleak, though, and you'll be thankful for what you have learned and the power that knowledge gives you.

It's impossible to predict every health scenario that can affect your loved one. Their dementia may progress at different speeds, and other physical and mental health problems may arise during that time. Advance care planning can't take care of all possibilities, but you can touch them in broad terms.

Your loved one may not always have access to the best treatments and professionals available, as everyone would have in an ideal world. But even if they can't recognize things around them, they are still human beings and need to be treated with dignity. Their wishes need to be respected, if it's their wish, for example, to stay at home instead of going to a care home or spending most of their time at a hospital.

FUTURE-PROOFING CARE STRATEGIES

Caregivers need to be informed about medical advancements and care techniques being developed. Establishing a supportive network, with each party doing their best, will get you better results than working by yourself. The support that you get from that network will make a difference during the many changes and shifts that dementia will bring.

You can start building your network by joining newsletters and reading journals about the subject. Education on dementia and elder care is more available now than ever on platforms such as Coursera or edX, as well as webinars and virtual conferences where you can connect with others. You can also use the internet to take part in support groups in online forums or social media platforms, like Facebook or LinkedIn.

It's important to see a geriatric specialist or neurologist at least two times a year to review your current plans. While you can get assistance from dementia care coaches or consultants, nothing beats the advice of a doctor who knows and has been following your loved one's case. The doctor/patient relationship is sacred and will guide you through the different types of healthcare systems.

The fact that plans change shouldn't discourage you from being careful and thorough when creating them. All strategies should be well thought out while leaving room for the changes that will inevitably come. Depending on the circumstances, you might have to review them more or less often. Even if things seem great, you should check everything at least bi-annually.

It's possible to benefit from the advice of people who have dealt with dementia, even if each case is different. Through their experience, you can develop your plans for the future, even if those plans have to change in the future. Then, with your own experience, you can help others and volunteer to participate in dementia research.

Academic research on dementia can always benefit from the experience of patients and caregivers. Clinical trials and studies can ask you to take cognitive and physical tests, as well as respond to questionnaires regarding the health of the patient with dementia. There are specific criteria to be part of this kind of research, and you may only participate in one research at a time.

Through research, academics can evaluate strategies to diagnose and treat dementia, both with and without medication, and test the effectiveness of medical devices used for exams. They are also interested in new ways of looking after caregivers. If you're interested in participating in such studies, look for the nearest Alzheimer's Disease Research Centers at nia.nih.gov or search the Alzheimer's Clinical Trials Finder at alzheimers.-gov/clinical-trials.

This kind of research can lead to significant changes in the way dementia is treated. One particular kind of medication is approved by the U.S. Food and Drug Administration (FDA) to treat dementia. It slows the progression of the disease, slowing the decline of the patient's brain and preserving their memory and cognition. These are based on anti-amyloids, which work to remove beta-amyloid, a substance that disrupts the connections between neurons. This treatment is more effective in the early stages of dementia, though results are still impressive in later stages.

Considering that dementia symptoms go beyond the loss of memory, it's important to take care of the behavioral and psychological issues related to the disease. We've already explored the importance of customizing a home to accommodate the patient's needs, as well as other important behavioral initiatives you must take. There are also specific drugs to take care of issues such as insomnia, anxiety, and agitation. There are also drugs known as atypical antipsychotics, which increase the flux of dopamine chemical pathways in the brain.

As with any drug, these should be used with caution, requiring the prescription and accompaniment of a health professional. Self-medication is a serious issue and can cause irreparable damage. As you talk to other caregivers, they may suggest a medication that has worked with their loved one, but every case is different, and only a professional can tell if that medication is going to work for your case.

LEGACY-BUILDING

Watching the progression of dementia in your loved one often feels like watching their essence going away. Their memories become confused; they gradually forget the names of people and things and start to feel like strangers in their own home. It's the hardest part of the whole process, but you can make it easier with a project to preserve the legacy of that person.

Each person has a set of values that they have lived by. Regardless of whether they're the CEO of a million-dollar company or the janitor at the local school—each person is unique and each life is an adventure! You can preserve the memory of that adventure and pass it on to future generations of the family in a way that will preserve what your loved one stands for!

Your loved one can record a video for a grandchild who, in the future, will have trouble remembering them. Memory can also be preserved in writing. The person with dementia can write a series of letters to the family, which should be open at specific times. It could be a collection of stories, a photo album, or a cookbook with their favorite recipes.

More than memories, it's important to pass values to the next generation. An elderly person has learned many lessons in their life, and it's important not to let those lessons fade away because of dementia. Making them part of family tradition will keep the flame alive and offer younger members someone to look up to.

A good tradition would be to take the loved one to a meaningful place on their birthday. Returning to this place after they have passed away is a more uplifting way of remembering them than visiting their grave.

There are many ways in which younger members of the family can be passed the torch. If your loved one plays an instrument, other members of the family could take lessons from them. Maybe they enjoy literature and could have reading sessions with their grandchildren regularly. This is the kind of activity that will keep them alive much after they shift their mortal coil.

INTERACTIVE ELEMENT

In this last interactive element session, we'll discuss the act of journaling. Taking a few minutes to write about your day and everything you've been through serves to drive away stress and anxiety, keep your mind focused, and help to reinterpret your journey.

Journaling is also valuable for caregivers, as it can help them get good sleep and heal from the hardships of each day. By putting your memories and thoughts on paper, you can stop dwelling on them and be able to move along to the next day. You don't have to produce fine prose, and nobody has to read it—it's just a way of coping with your thoughts.

If you have trouble starting your journaling or feel that there's nothing interesting about your life, you can always try journal prompts. These are simple questions that serve to ignite your ideas so that you can get in the right rhythm. Here are some examples:

- What new thing did you do today?
- Mention one thing you think you could be better at.

- Of all the meals you had recently, which one did you enjoy the most?
- List three things that happened today that made you happy.
- If you had to learn something new, what would it be?
- Is there a goal you haven't accomplished yet, and how could you accomplish it?
- Would you say today was a good or bad day? Why?
- Did you do something today that would make someone proud?
- Do you still live in the same place you grew up in? If not, when was the last time you've been there?
- Is your life better now than it was five years ago?
- Write about the last film or a book you read.

Another good idea is to start a journal with your loved one, encouraging them to recall their youth and the people they've met. For that, Samuels (2023a) offers the following prompts:

- Do you know the history of your family name, crest, or origin?
- What do you remember about your parents and grandparents? This is a special opportunity to learn more about family members you didn't have the chance to meet.
- What were your children like growing up? Do they have any funny or embarrassing stories about Mom or Dad?
- What did you and your siblings do for fun? Maybe straight-laced Aunt Ruth was a huge troublemaker back in the day!
- How did you meet your spouse? Was it love at first sight or an uphill battle? What was the wedding like?
- What are the most rewarding things about getting older? Is it a lifetime of knowledge? The senior discount

at the movie theatre?

- What are the most important lessons you've learned in your life? Ask to hear the stories behind those lessons.
- Who has influenced you the most? Thank your loved one for the ways they've influenced your life so far.
- What life advice would you pass along? Take this answer to heart.
- If you could go back to any age, what would it be? Would they stay the age they are now or go back? How far back? What was life like at that time?

What differentiates a journal from a memoir is that the memoir is typically written a long time after the events took place, while the journal is written as things happen. That means you write today without knowing what's going to happen tomorrow. Because of that, journals make a fascinating read if you check them years later.

You may also find it hard to understand certain ideas and emotions. Not every journal is written to be read afterward. Some people prefer to destroy them once they're complete as a way of cutting ties with the past that they represent.

ERIC'S STORY

Ever since Eric can remember, he has seen the accordion on his Uncle Joe's shelf. It's not hidden behind a glass, nor is it on a high shelf, but he's still afraid to touch it. When he was little, he thought it was a small piano because of the keys. As he grew up, he learned what an accordion was. He also learned that this accordion belonged to his grandfather, who died when he was two. Eric has no recollection of Grandpa, though he has seen a lot of pictures of him. In those, he looked like a funny old man who loved to play music. Eric wished there was a recording of it.

Uncle Joe has a big house and always hosts family parties. It's a big family, the kind that gets together for every birthday. When Eric turned fourteen, he decided to ask the family why Uncle Joe had the accordion. They told him that Grandpa had dementia for the last four years of his life and didn't leave a will. Uncle Joe was the first one to claim the instrument.

Out of curiosity, Eric started watching a lot of videos of people playing the accordion. He found the instrument fascinating, with all its complexities. One day, he asked his dad if he could take accordion lessons. They looked up prices online and found out how expensive an accordion can be.

"Can't I get the one from Grandpa?" he asked. "It's just sitting at Uncle Joe's house."

A year passes. They're once again having a party at Uncle Joe's, but this time, the accordion isn't on the shelf. Eric plays the instrument for everyone, and they say that it's like seeing Grandpa coming back to life.

SEGUE

In this chapter, we've seen what a progressive disease is and how it operates inside a person's mind. As dementia progresses, our strategies need to change, which is why it's important to have built a solid foundation during the early stages of the disease. The key is to always stay informed, know the territory you're stepping into, and be aware of the latest advances in the field of medicine.

As we arrive at the end of this book, I hope you have acquired useful knowledge that will make a difference. Now that you know how to manage finances and legalities, embrace technology, and take care of yourself, I believe you have become a better caregiver.

AFTERWORD

Dementia is a part of the lives of millions of people around the world. In most cases, people are caught off guard and must learn how to deal with it as they go along. When I sat down to start writing this book, I promised myself I wouldn't try to make the journey of a caregiver sound easier than it is. I didn't want to write a book full of motivational messages such as "You can do this!" nor did I want to write a horror book showing this journey as something that's going to ruin you. There are plenty of books on that already. So why write another one?

Caregivers can't afford to live in a make-believe world. Because of that, I decided to write a book about how it is to be a caregiver that deals with real adult issues, such as finances, legal matters, and dealing with medical professionals. More than motivation, I wanted to give you real tools that you can use in your daily life.

We live in a world where information is available to anyone. However, it's not always easy to find and interpret that information. My job here was to select all the information that I wished I had when I first started my journey and to present it to you in a way that makes sense. This way, you don't have to spend your time looking for it and can focus on what matters most: your loved one.

Every moment you spend with your loved one with dementia will make a difference. A difference in their mind, for they will be able to remember you longer, and also in your mind, for you will have moments to cherish long after they're gone. By following the advice I included here, you will be able to optimize every hour of your day.

If you enjoyed this book, please leave a review—it makes all the difference in the world, and it helps me to continue producing this kind of content. I also suggest that you present this book to people in your circle who are also dealing with a loved one with dementia. They, too, can benefit from the knowledge that I included here, and that will improve everyone's journey! Also, tell them about my other book, *Compassionate Care: Navigating Dementia Together*, for a complete experience.

Thank you for reading! Let this book guide you to moments of joy and peace with your loved one. And don't forget to share your story. Your insights could make a difference for others who are struggling with caregiving. Stand tall as a beacon within the dementia care community—your voice, your experience, and your compassion can transform lives.

REQUEST FOR REVIEW

At the conclusion of the book, I want to say **Thank You!** for choosing Compassionate Care: A Practical Guide for Dementia Caregiving. I would be deeply grateful if you would share a review. Your opinion matters so much. By scanning the relevant QR Code with your phone or tablet, or by using the appropriate link below you can easily share your honest review and help spread the important information in this book.

Your words play an important role, helping others learn and maybe changing their lives, and guiding me to better share what I have learned about caregiving. Your personal contribution is part of navigating together.

To leave a review, scan the QR code using your phone or tablet, or enter the link in your browser.

Amazon USA

CompassionateCare.fyi/leave-review-USA

Amazon CANADA

CompassionateCare.fyi/leave-review-CANADA

Amazon UNITED KINGDOM

CompassionateCare.fyi/leave-review-UK

If you haven't already, you can request the free Compassionate Care gifts which were mentioned in the beginning of the book.

GLOSSARY

ADLs (Activities of Daily Living): Basic essential tasks that need to be fulfilled to maintain one's basic needs, such as eating, bathing, toileting, dressing, grooming, and transferring.

Advance Directive (AD): A document in which the dementia patient explains their wishes and directs how their medical treatment should function. The AD is written and signed while the person is still in possession of their mental faculties.

Alzheimer's Disease: The most common cause of dementia in the US, Alzheimer's is a progressive disease that affects memory, thinking, and behavior. Alzheimer's development is often slow, and with time can make common daily tasks impossible.

Alzheimer's Disease Programs Initiative (ADPI): A federal program created to assist those with dementia and their families.

Apathy: Absence of interest, enthusiasm, or concern.

Appropriate care: The type of care that's selected among all existing types as the one that can offer the most benefit to a specific dementia patient.

Assessment: The ongoing process of evaluating the person's capacity of living independently and how much help they require.

Assistive Technology: Electronic devices that help one's memory.

Behavioral and Psychological Symptoms of Dementia (BPSD): Disruptive actions from the dementia patient caused by an unmet need. They can manifest as aggressions, compulsions, paranoia, and other unwanted behaviors.

Beneficiary: The person who enjoys the benefits of a grant.

Care Plan: An outline detailing the care goals for people with dementia by analyzing their physical and psychosocial strengths and weaknesses. This document needs to be developed together with the patients, their families, and any medical specialist who is taking care of the case.

Challenging Behavior: Harsh behavior from the dementia patient, which has the potential to harm or disturb those around them, especially their family and caregivers. This behavior may be born from the frustration of the dementia patient to communicate with those around them.

Cognition: The ensemble of perceptions that allow us to rationalize and understand ourselves and the world around us.

Delusion: A fixation that an illogical and false situation is true. Delusions often occur when the person mixes and distorts things that actually happen.

Dementia: A term that encompasses several symptoms connected with the loss of memory and cognition, which can be caused by a disease such as Alzheimer's or by a physical injury to the brain.

Depression: An unnatural feeling of sadness and hopelessness that's different from normal daily changes of mood. Depression happens for no apparent reason, though it can be increased by stress, abuse, drug and alcohol abuse, or the loss of a loved one.

Do Not Resuscitate (DNR): A code that allows the patient to die of natural causes instead of keeping them alive artificially through medical instruments.

Eldercare Attorney: An attorney who specializes in dealing with elderly clients.

Experiential self: The part of our consciousness that is aware of the world around us and absorbs its stimuli through our five physical senses.

Frontal Lobe: The part of the brain behind the forehead that controls emotions, personality, and cognition.

Frontotemporal dementia: A rare type of dementia that affects the frontal lobe of people between their thirties and sixties, affecting their social behavior and capacity of speech. People with frontotemporal dementia are often agitated and incur obsessive and repetitive behavior, but their memory isn't affected during the first stages of the disease.

GPS Tracker: A device that uses satellite technology to determine a person's location.

Grantor: The creator and founder of a trust.

Guardian: A person appointed to make decisions on behalf of the patient with dementia who can no longer make those decisions themselves.

Hallucination: A visual, auditory, or olfactory perception of something that's not there. Alzheimer's patients are prone to have hallucinations.

HIPAA: A document through which the dementia patient consents a third party to use or disclose their protected health information

Hippocampus: Part of the brain that generates short-term memory and emotions.

History: Medical and psycho-social history serve to detail previous treatments and incidents that the person has gone through, as to facilitate further treatment.

Incontinence: Incapacity of controlling bladder and bowel functions. This is a common symptom in Alzheimer's patients and can be treated in its early stages, though the use of geriatric diapers may become necessary.

Instrumental Activities of Daily Living (IADLs): Home management activities that improve people's lives in a community, though they are not as crucial as the ADLs. It includes housekeeping, financial management, preparing meals, getting around in a vehicle or public transportation, managing medicines, etc.

Intuitive thought processes: Thought process that happens in the right side of the brain and which happens spontaneously and instantaneously, without requiring effort. Through the intuitive process, we get feelings, impressions, and instinctive responses, even if those contradict our rational feelings. Intuitive thought processes are fueled by our past experiences, and they allow us to enjoy art and beauty.

Irrevocable Trust: A trust in which the terms cannot be modified.

Level of Care: Divided into mild (or "early"), moderate (or "middle"), and severe (or "late") this term reflects the amount of care that a person needs at a given point of their dementia treatment. The level of care is usually low at the moment of the diagnosis, but symptoms get worse as the disease progresses, and it's important to know when and how to get help.

Living Will: A document written and signed by a dementia patient after the diagnosis, but while they're still in control of their cognitive abilities. Through the living will, the dementia patient states their medical wishes and makes provisions for legal matters that may arise when they are not fully conscious anymore.

Long-Term Memory: Memory that can be stored indefinitely, holding an unlimited amount of information.

Medicaid: A federal and state program covering medical costs for those with limited resources.

Medicare: A government national health insurance program.

Mild Cognitive Impairment (MCI): A cognitive problem that can be perceived but is not strong enough to have a harmful impact on a person's life.

Mindfulness: The basic human ability of being conscious of the world around you, being present, and perceiving things around you. It can be achieved through meditation and mental exercises.

Mindlessness: The opposite of mindfulness—being unaware of what you're doing, making unconscious decisions because your mind is wandering.

Motion Activated Lights: Electric lights are activated by a motion sensor without the need to press a switch.

National Family Caregiver Support Program (NFCSP): Federal program created to assist family members that serve as informal caregivers for patients with dementia.

Neurodegenerative: Diseases that affect the structure and functioning of the brain tissue. Neurodegenerative diseases are more common in the elderly but can show up in younger people.

Neurology: A medical field that deals with the nervous system.

Occipital Lobe: Part of the brain that controls sight and the capacity to recognize things. Located at the lower rear of the bran.

Paranoia: An acute feeling of suspicion without rational reasoning behind it.

Parietal Lobes: Part of the brain responsible for touch, pressure, pain, temperature, and taste. Located at the upper rear of the brain.

Parkinson's Disease: Neurological disorder that interferes with muscle, affecting gait and facial features, as well as causing tremors. Parkinson's usually occurs during the early sixties and moves slowly and progressively, and can cause symptoms of dementia.

Pathology: Field of medicine that studies diseases, establishing its causes, symptoms, and effects, by examining their impacts on the body.

Perception: Recognizing external stimuli through the five senses and interpreting them through an unconscious memory association.

Power of Attorney: Authority to make legal decisions on behalf of a person who cannot take them by themselves.

Psychosocial: The psychological and social aspects related to a person's behavior.

Psychotropic Drugs: Drugs that have an effect on the brain, influencing a person's mental health. They can be antidepressants, anxiolytics, tranquilizers, and other drugs that have an effect on the patient's emotions and behavior.

Rational Thought Processes: These processes happen on the left side of the brain and are responsible for making methodical choices, making interpretations, prioritizing actions and information, and following steps to achieve a goal. This kind of thought requires effort and can tell us if we are having proper behavior during a situation and how to act from there.

Removable Trust: A trust whose terms can be changed at any time.

Reverse Mortgage: A home loan that isn't charged while the person continues to live in the house.

Smart Home: A house where most functioning devices can be controlled remotely.

Social Security Disability Insurance (SSDI): Federal insurance program managed by the Social Security Administration that offers assistance to those who are unable to work.

Sundowning Syndrome: Sensation of disorientation and irritability that some people with dementia have when the sun goes down at the end of the day. Its causes are not clear but could have to do with the change in the environment or the feeling of tiredness.

Temporal Lobes: Part of the brain responsible for audition, also connected with memory, language, emotion, interpretation, and learning and located above the ears.

Trust: A legal entity that manages a person's organization's funds. It allows those funds to be moved between the interested parties without intermediation from the government.

Trustee: The person who manages a grant according to the grantor's wishes and instructions.

Vascular Dementia: This type of dementia caused by several small strokes, which are often not perceived, but can have an impact on the brain.

Wandering: Moving around aimlessly without a goal or direction, which can bring a person with dementia to exhaustion or take them to a place where their security is at risk. It's possible to wander safely if there's an appropriate space for that, such as a garden or a backyard.

Ward of Court: A person appointed by the court to manage the affairs of a dementia patient who has been declared legally incapable of doing that themselves

REFERENCES

About me. (2020, August 30). The Other Side of Dying. https://dahliasfordaddy.com/about-me/

Ackerman, C. E., MA. (2023, April 26). *87 self-reflection questions for introspection.* PositivePsychology.com. https://positivepsychology.com/introspection-self-reflection/

Activities for people with dementia: 30 expert tips for daily activities and routines. (2023, December 13). Careforth. https://careforth.com/blog/activities-for-dementia-patients-50-tips-and-ideas-to-keep-patients-with-dementia-engaged/

Advance care planning: Advance directives for health care. (n.d.). National Institute on Aging. https://www.nia.nih.gov/health/advance-care-planning/advance-care-planning-advance-directives-health-care

Advance care planning for patients with Alzheimer's disease – Advance care planning (ACP) decisions. (n.d.). ACP Decisions. https://www.acpdecisions.org/advance-care-planning-for-patients-with-alzheimers-disease/

Advance directives for patients with Alzheimer's. (n.d.). VITAS Healthcare. https://www.vitas.com/hospice-and-palliative-care-basics/end-of-life-care-planning/living-wills-and-advance-directives/advance-directives-for-patients-with-alzheimers

Allen, R. S. (2009). The Legacy Project Intervention to Enhance Meaningful Family Interactions: case examples. *Clinical Gerontologist, 32*(2), 164–176. https://doi.org/10.1080/07317110802677005

Allen, R. S., Hilgeman, M. M., Ege, M. A., Shuster, J. L., & Burgio, L. D. (2008). Legacy activities as interventions approaching the end of life. *Journal of Palliative Medicine,* 11(7), 1029–1038. https://doi.org/10.1089/jpm.2007.0294

Alzheimers and dementia care. (2018, January 9). VeteranAid. https://www.veteranaid.org/alzheimers-demnetia.php#google_vignette

Alzheimer's caregiving: Caring for yourself. (n.d.). National Institute on Aging. https://www.nia.nih.gov/health/alzheimers-caregiving-caring-yourself

Automatic pill dispenser - How the hero dispenser works! (n.d.). Hero. https://hero-health.com/our-product/

Baig, E. C. (2023, May 1). *5 Ways tech can help caregivers of dementia patients.* AARP. https://www.aarp.org/home-family/personal-technology/info-2023/dementia-caregiver-technology.html

Bailey, M. (2021, September 26). *The 3 roles in a they're important to understand before sitting down with your estate planning attorney.* Michael Bailey Law, LLC.

https://michaelbaileylawllc.com/the-3-roles-in-a-trust-and-why-theyre-important-to-understand-before-sitting-down-with-your-estate-planning-attorney/

Basu, N. (2021, November 11). *Using a revocable living trust to prepare for assisted living and dementia*. Norton Basu LLP. https://www.nortonbasu.com/blog/2020/09/revocable-living-trust-assisted-living-dementia/

Be a healthy caregiver. (n.d.). Alzheimer's Disease and Dementia. https://www.alz.org/help-support/caregiving/caregiver-health/be_a_healthy_caregiver

Behavior & personality changes. (n.d.). Memory and Aging Center. https://memory.ucsf.edu/caregiving-support/behavior-personality-changes

Black, A. (2022, December 22). *Irrevocable trusts*. Vertical Estate Planning. https://verticalestateplanning.com/add-page/irrevocable-trusts/

Bosisio, F., Sterie, A., Truchard, E. R., & Jox, R. J. (2021). Implementing advance care planning in early dementia care: results and insights from a pilot intervention trial. *BMC Geriatrics, 21*. https://doi.org/10.1186/s12877-021-02529-8

Brodaty, H., & Donkin, M. (2009). Family caregivers of people with dementia. *Dialogues in Clinical Neuroscience*. https://doi.org/10.31887/dcns.2009.11.2/hbrodaty

Caitlin. (2020, November 17). *Best practices: Zoom video calls & dementia*. Alzheimer's San Diego. https://www.alzsd.org/best-practices-zoom-video-calls-dementia/

Can someone with dementia make a will? (n.d.). Alzheimer's Society. https://www.alzheimers.org.uk/get-support/publications-and-fact-sheets/dementia-together-magazine/can-someone-dementia-make-will

Caregiver stress. (n.d.). Alzheimer's Association. https://www.alz.org/help-support/caregiving/caregiver-health/caregiver-stress

Caregiver stress: Tips for taking care of yourself. (2023, August 9). Mayo Clinic. https://www.mayoclinic.org/healthy-lifestyle/stress-management/in-depth/caregiver-stress/art-20044784

Caregiving at home: A guide to community resources. (2021, June 4). Family Caregiver Alliance. https://www.caregiver.org/resource/caregiving-home-guide-community-resources/

Chiong, W., Tsou, A. Y., Simmons, Z., Bonnie, R. J., Russell, J. A., & Ethics, L. (2021). Ethical Considerations in Dementia Diagnosis and care. *Neurology, 97(2)*, 80–89. https://doi.org/10.1212/wnl.0000000000012079

Cobb, D. (2022, April 5). *Paying for Alzheimer's care: Financial help, costs & care options*. Paying for Senior Care. https://www.payingforseniorcare.com/memory-care

Conservatorship and guardianship. (2021, December 30). Family Caregiver Alliance. https://www.caregiver.org/resource/conservatorship-and-guardianship/

Covering the costs of long-term dementia care. (n.d.). Healthy You. https://www.riversideonline.com/patients-and-visitors/healthy-you-blog/blog/c/covering-the-costs-of-long-term-dementia-care

Cost of care survey. (2023). Genworth. https://www.genworth.com/aging-and-you/finances/cost-of-care.html

Creating meaningful interactions with a loved one with memory loss. (2022, May 3). Highgate Senior Living. https://blog.highgateseniorliving.com/creating-meaningful-interactions-with-a-loved-one-with-memory-loss

Cutner, L. &. (2023, August 10). Asset protection is imperative for Alzheimer's & dementia patients. Lamson & Cutner. https://www.cutner.com/asset-protection-is-imperative-for-alzheimers-dementia-patients/

Daugherty, G. (2022, August 27). Asset Protection Trusts: help for seniors. Investopedia. https://www.investopedia.com/articles/personal-finance/110514/asset-protection-trusts-help-seniors.asp

Davis, J. (2023, October 31). Understanding the costs of dementia care. North River Home Care. https://www.northriverhc.com/understanding-the-costs-of-dementia-care/

de Cervantes, M. (n.d.). Miguel de Cervantes quotes. BrainyQuote. https://www.brainyquote.com/quotes/miguel_de_cervantes_131381

Decision-making and respecting independence. (n.d.). Alzheimer Society of Canada. https://alzheimer.ca/en/help-support/im-caring-person-living-dementia/providing-day-day-care/decision-making-respecting

Delaney, J. R. (2022, May 10). How to set up your smart home: a beginner's guide. PCMAG. https://www.pcmag.com/how-to/how-to-set-up-your-smart-home-a-beginners-guide

Dementia care costs by state: An overview of costs, types of dementia care, and the cost of dementia care by state. (2023, November 26). Careforth. https://careforth.com/blog/dementia-care-costs-by-state-an-overview-of-costs-types-of-dementia-care-and-the-cost-of-dementia-care-by-state/

Dementia insights: The validation method for dementia care. Practical Neurology. https://practicalneurology.com/articles/2022-mar-apr/dementia-insights-the-validation-method-for-dementia-care

Dementia care practice recommendations for professionals working in a home setting. (2009). Alzheimer's Association. https://www.alz.org/national/documents/phase_4_home_care_recs.pdf

Dementia may cause problems with money management years before diagnosis. (2021, January 14). National Institute on Aging. https://www.nia.nih.gov/news/dementia-may-cause-problems-money-management-years-before-diagnosis

Dementia-friendly environments. (n.d.). Social Care Institute for Excellence. https://www.scie.org.uk/dementia/supporting-people-with-dementia/dementia-friendly-environments/

Dementia - behaviour changes. (n.d.). Better Health Channel. https://www.betterhealth.vic.gov.au/health/conditionsandtreatments/dementia-behaviour-changes

Desai, N. (2023, December 8). *Useful dementia apps for seniors and their caregivers.* A Place for Mom. https://www.aplaceformom.com/caregiver-resources/articles/dementia-apps

Dhue, S., & Epperson, S. (2023, August 31). *How to prevent burnout and financial stress when caring for an elderly parent or relative.* CNBC. https://www.cnbc.com/2023/08/29/preventing-burnout-financial-stress-when-caring-for-elderly-relatives.html

Dieleman, J. L. (2022). Global and regional spending on dementia care from 2000–2019 and expected future health spending scenarios from 2020–2050: An economic modelling exercise. *EClinicalMedicine.* https://www.ncbi.nlm.nih.gov/pmc/articles/PMC8921543/

Digital technology for the family caregiver. (2021, December 31). Family Caregiver Alliance. https://www.caregiver.org/resource/digital-technology-family-caregiver/

DOesLongterm care insurance cover memory care? A comprehensive guide. (n.d.). The National Council on Aging. https://www.ncoa.org/article/does-long-term-care-insurance-cover-memory-care-a-comprehensive-guide

Duties and responsibilities of a trustee in estate planning. (n.d.). EstatePlanning.com. https://www.estateplanning.com/duties-and-responsibilities-of-a-trustee

Eason, H. (2023, November 29). *Everything you need to know about the cost of memory care: a State-by-State guide.* A Place For Mom. https://www.aplaceformom.com/caregiver-resources/articles/cost-of-memory-care

Ferraz, M. (2022, April 5). *Cracking the secrets of memoir writing: Ferraz, Matt: Books.* https://www.amazon.com/Cracking-Secrets-Memoir-Writing-Ferraz-ebook/dp/B09XBLLBKC/

Feurich, V. (2023, April 20). *7 tips for building an effective dementia care support team.* Positive Approach to Care. https://teepasnow.com/blog/7-tips-for-building-an-effective-dementia-care-support-team/

15 Caregiver Stress Management. (n.d.). A Train Education. https://www.a-trainceu.com/content/15-caregiver-stress-management

15 meaningful activities for dementia patients.(2023, November 3). Senior Services of America. https://seniorservicesofamerica.com/blog/15-meaningful-activities-for-dementia-patients/

50 activities. (n.d.). Alzheimer's Association. https://www.alz.org/help-support/resources/kids-teens/50-activities

Finances and Caregiving: A guide to navigating financial challenges. (2023, October 5). Linkedin. https://www.linkedin.com/pulse/finances-caregiving-guide-navigating-financial-challenges/

Financial planning. (n.d.). Alzheimer's Association. https://www.alz.org/help-support/i-have-alz/plan-for-your-future/financial_planning

5 money management tips for family caregivers. (n.d.). Fulton Bank. https://www.-

fultonbank.com/Education-Center/Family-and-Finance/5-Financial-Tips-for-Caregivers

5 smart tips for hiring an elder law Attorney. (2023, March 29). DailyCaring. https://dailycaring.com/how-to-find-an-elder-law-attorney-you-can-trust/

5 things to consider when tailoring your home environment for a Loved one with Dementia. (2019, December 2). Project We Forgot. https://projectweforgot.com/articles/5-things-to-consider-when-tailoring-your-home-environment-for-a-loved-one-with-dementia/

Future proofing dementia care. (n.d.) Care Talk. https://www.caretalk.co.uk/opinion/future-proofing-dementia-care/

Gaunt, A. (2023, July 3). 9 Lifesaving location devices for dementia patients. Our Parents. https://www.ourparents.com/products-for-seniors/location-devices-dementia

Getting financial help for dementia & Alzheimer's care. (2023, February 15). Dementia Care Central. https://www.dementiacarecentral.com/financial-assistance/

Graham, B. (n.d.). Billy Graham quotes. BrainyQuote. https://www.brainyquote.com/quotes/billy_graham_626354

Guardianship & conservatorship of incapacitated persons. (n.d.) Commonwealth of Massachusetts. https://www.mass.gov/guardianship-conservatorship-of-incapacitated-persons

Guide: Navigating long term care insurance. (n.d.). Home Instead. https://www.homeinstead.com/care-resources/care-planning/guide-navigating-long-term-care-insurance/

Guide to choosing a GPS tracker for dementia care. (2022, October 21). Tack GPS. https://www.tackgps.app/post/guide-to-choosing-a-gps-tracker-for-dementia-care

Hasson, J. (2023, September 5). A legal checklist for family caregivers. AARP. https://www.aarp.org/caregiving/financial-legal/info-2020/caregivers-legal-checklist.html

The health plan categories: Bronze, silver, gold & platinum. (n.d.). HealthCare.gov. https://www.healthcare.gov/choose-a-plan/plans-categories/

How can I find an attorney who specializes in elder law? (2022, August 18). Consumer Financial Protection Bureau. https://www.consumerfinance.gov/ask-cfpb/how-can-i-find-an-attorney-who-specializes-in-elder-law-en-1159/

How do you do a video call with your doctor? (2022, April 6). Sharp HealthCare. https://www.sharp.com/health-news/how-to-prep-for-your-virtual-care-visit

How much care will you need? (n.d.) ACL Administration for Community Living. https://acl.gov/ltc/basic-needs/how-much-care-will-you-need

How to apply for Medicaid (n.d.) DSHS. https://www.dshs.wa.gov/altsa/home-and-community-services/how-apply-medicaid

How to apply for Medicaid. (2019, November 12). Medicare Interactive. https://www.medicareinteractive.org/get-answers/cost-saving-programs-for-people-with-medicare/medicare-and-medicaid/how-to-apply-for-medicaid

How to make your home dementia friendly. (2023, August 18). NHS.uk. https://www.nhs.uk/conditions/dementia/living-with-dementia/home-environment/

How to prepare for a video call with a doctor. (2021, September 22). My Pill & More. https://mypillandmore.com/2021/09/04/how-to-prepare-for-a-video-call-with-a-doctor/

Huang, S. (2022). Depression among caregivers of patients with dementia: Associative factors and management approaches. *World Journal of Psychiatry*, 12(1), 59–76. https://doi.org/10.5498/wjp.v12.i1.59

In focus: Spreading innovative approaches to dementia care. (2017, December 20). Commonwealth Fund. https://www.commonwealthfund.org/publications/2017/dec/focus-spreading-innovative-approaches-dementia-care

Lasting power of attorney for people with dementia. (n.d.). Alzheimer's Society. https://www.alzheimers.org.uk/get-support/legal-financial/lasting-power-attorney

Law, N. F. a. A. (2022, December 30). *6 qualities to look for in elder law attorneys.* Neuberger, Griggs, Sweet & Froehle, LLP. https://www.watertownlaw.com/6-qualities-to-look-for-in-elder-law-attorneys

Leaving your legacy. (n.d.). Alzheimer's Disease and Dementia. https://www.alz.org/help-support/i-have-alz/live-well/leaving-your-legacy

Legal documents. (n.d.). Alzheimer's Disease and Dementia. https://www.alz.org/help-support/caregiving/financial-legal-planning/legal-documents

Legal planning. (n.d.). Alzheimer's Disease and Dementia. https://www.alz.org/help-support/i-have-alz/plan-for-your-future/legal_-planning

Leveraging content to support virtual care. (n.d.). Healthwise. https://www.healthwise.org/blog/leveraging-content.aspx

Li, J., Wang, S., & Nicholas, L. H. (2022a). Management of financial assets by older adults with and without dementia or other cognitive impairments. *JAMA Network Open*, 5(9), e2231436. https://doi.org/10.1001/jamanetworkopen.2022.31436

Livingston, G., Huntley, J., Sommerlad, A., Ames, D., Ballard, C., Banerjee, S., Brayne, C., Burns, A., Cohen-Mansfield, J., Cooper, C., Costafreda, S. G., Dias, A., Fox, N. C., Gitlin, L. N., Howard, R., Kales, H. C., Kivimäki, M., Larson, E. B., Ogunniyi, A., . . . Mukadam, N. (2020). Dementia prevention, intervention, and care: 2020 report of the Lancet Commission. *The Lancet*, 396(10248), 413–446. https://doi.org/10.1016/s0140-6736(20)30367-6

Lundberg, A. (2023, November 6). *20 Engaging activities for people with dementia at home*. A Place For Mom. https://www.aplaceformom.com/caregiver-resources/articles/dementia-activities

Make a power of attorney for a loved one with dementia. (2023, November 27). Rocket Lawyer. https://www.rocketlawyer.com/family-and-personal/estate-planning/power-of-attorney/legal-guide/obtain-a-durable-poa-for-a-parent-with-dementia-alzheimers

Making financial plans after a diagnosis of dementia. (2016).Alzheimer Association. https://www.alz.org/national/documents/brochure_moneymatters.pdf

Managing finances for people with dementia. (n.d.). Alzheimer's Society. https://www.alzheimers.org.uk/get-support/daily-living/making-decisions-and-managing-difficult-situations/finances

Managing money problems for people with dementia. (n.d.). National Institute on Aging. https://www.nia.nih.gov/health/managing-money-problems-people-dementia

Managing the financial risks of dementia and cognitive decline. (2023, November 1). RBC Wealth Management. https://www.rbcwealthmanagement.com/en-us/insights/the-financial-impact-of-dementia

Marson, D. C. (2013). Clinical and ethical aspects of financial capacity in Dementia: a commentary. *American Journal of Geriatric Psychiatry, 21*(4), 382–390. https://doi.org/10.1016/j.jagp.2013.01.033

Medicare. (2023, September 27). Nacional Council on Aging. https://www.alz.org/help-support/caregiving/financial-legal-planning/medicare

Memory aids and tools. (2021, August 11). Alzheimer's Society. https://www.alzheimers.org.uk/get-support/staying-independent/memory-aids-and-tools

Memory loss: Remember to plan. (2023, August 22). Fiduciary Trust. https://www.-fiduciary-trust.com/insights/memory-loss-remember-to-plan/

Mitchell, S. L., Black, B. S., Ersek, M., Hanson, L. C., Miller, S. C., Sachs, G. A., Teno, J. M., & Morrison, R. S. (2012). Advanced Dementia: state of the art and priorities for the next decade. *Annals of Internal Medicine, 156*(1_Part_1), 45. https://doi.org/10.7326/0003-4819-156-1-201201030-00008

Moeller, P. (2018, January 10). *10 questions to ask before hiring an elder care attorney*. PBS NewsHour. https://www.pbs.org/newshour/economy/making-sense/10-questions-to-ask-before-hiring-an-elder-care-attorney

Monekosso, D. (n.d.). *Truly smart homes could help dementia patients live independently*. The Conversation. https://theconversation.com/truly-smart-homes-could-help-dementia-patients-live-independently-123104

National Academies of Sciences, Engineering, and Medicine. (2021) *Reducing the impact of dementia in America: A decadal survey of the behavioral and social sciences*. NIH. https://www.ncbi.nlm.nih.gov/books/NBK574334/

National family caregiver support. (n.d.). Maryland Department of Aging. https://aging.maryland.gov/Pages/national-family-caregiver-support.aspx

National family caregiver support program. (n.d.). Administration for Community Living http://acl.gov/programs/support-caregivers/national-family-caregiver-support-program

9 steps on how to create a will. (n.d.). Empower. https://www.empower.com/the-currency/life/9-things-you-need-to-know-about-creating-a-will

Nursing home costs by state and region. (2022, March 4). American Council of Aging. https://www.medicaidplanningassistance.org/nursing-home-costs/

Osborne, M. (2022, September 20). *How to apply for guardianship of a parent with dementia?* Your Dementia Therapist. https://yourdementiatherapist.com/alzheimers-dementia/caregiving/guardianship-for-adults/

Palmer, P. (n.d.). *Parker Palmer quotes.* Goodreads. https://www.goodreads.com/quotes/1335101-self-care-is-never-a-selfish-act---it-is-simply

Participating in Alzheimer's disease and related dementia research. (n.d.). National Institute on Aging. https://www.nia.nih.gov/health/participating-alzheimers-disease-and-related-dementias-research

Paying for care. (n.d.). Alzheimer's Disease and Dementia. https://www.alz.org/help-support/caregiving/financial-legal-planning/paying-for-care

Piers, R., Albers, G., Gilissen, J., De Lepeleire, J., Steyaert, J., Van Mechelen, W., Steeman, E., Dillen, L., Vanden Berghe, P., & Van Den Block, L. (2018). Advance care planning in dementia: recommendations for healthcare professionals. *BMC Palliative Care,* 17(1). https://doi.org/10.1186/s12904-018-0332-2

Planning after a dementia diagnosis. (n.d.). Alzheimers.gov. https://www.alzheimers.gov/life-with-dementia/planning-for-future#tips-for-planning

Planning ahead for legal matters. (n.d.). Alzheimer's Disease and Dementia. https://www.alz.org/help-support/caregiving/financial-legal-planning/planning-ahead-for-legal-matters

Planning for care costs. (n.d.). Alzheimer's Association. https://www.alz.org/help-support/caregiving/financial-legal-planning/planning-for-care-costs

Porteri, C. (2018). Advance directives as a tool to respect patients' values and preferences: discussion on the case of Alzheimer's disease. *BMC Medical Ethics,* 19(1). https://doi.org/10.1186/s12910-018-0249-6

Power of attorney may fall short for those with Alzheimer's. (n.d.). Carolina Family Estate Planning. https://www.carolinafep.com/library/power-of-attorney-may-fall-short-for-individuals-with-alzheimer-s-or-dementia.cfm

Preparing for a virtual visit. (2023, July 31). Telehealth. https://telehealth.hhs.gov/patients/preparing-for-a-video-visit

Progression of dementia. (n.d.). Dementia Australia. https://www.dementia.org.au/about-dementia/what-is-dementia/progression-of-dementia

Randolph, M., JD. (2020, August 11). *Estate planning when you're concerned about dementia*. Nolo. https://www.nolo.com/legal-encyclopedia/estate-planning-when-you-re-concerned-about-dementia.html

Reducing the impact of dementia in America. (2021). National Academies Press eBooks. https://doi.org/10.17226/26175

Resources for caregivers of people with Alzheimer's disease and related dementias. (n.d.). Alzheimer's.Gov. https://www.alzheimers.gov/life-with-dementia/resources-caregivers

Roles, responsibilities, and duties of parties to a trust. (2017, March 20). Krasa Law, Inc. https://krasalaw.com/2017/03/20/the-roles-responsibilities-and-duties-of-parties-to-a-trust/

Ross, E., Levy, C., Ty, D., Altimus, C., & Super, N. (2022). *Roadmap for investment in dementia care*. Milken Institute. https://milkeninstitute.org/sites/default/files/2022-03/MI_DementiaCare_022822_final.pdf

Roth, D. L., Brown, S. L., Rhodes, J., & Haley, W. E. (2018). Reduced mortality rates among caregivers: Does family caregiving provide a stress-buffering effect? *Psychology and Aging*, 33(4), 619–629. https://doi.org/10.1037/pag0000224

Rsizelove. (2023, March 15). *From a dementia caregiver: 10 tips for self-care*. Hope-Health. https://www.hopehealthco.org/blog/from-a-dementia-caregiver-10-tips-for-self-care/

Rubin, H. (2023, April 30). *Financial vs. medical power of attorney: What's the difference?* Investopedia. https://www.investopedia.com/articles/managing-wealth/042216/medical-vs-financial-power-attorney-reasons-separate-them.asp

Sageage. (2021, October 26). *The challenges of changing environments for your loved one with dementia (and how to overcome them)*. Bridges by EPOCH. https://www.bridgesbyepoch.com/2020/02/17/challenges-changing-environments-your-loved-one-dementia-and-how/

Samuels, C. (2023a, May 5). *20 questions to ask elderly loved ones to connect and reminisce*. A Place For Mom. https://www.aplaceformom.com/caregiver-resources/articles/engaging-questions

Samuels, C. (2023b, November 8). *Does insurance cover memory care? A detailed look at coverage and options*. A Place For Mom. https://www.aplaceformom.com/caregiver-resources/articles/does-insurance-cover-memory-care

Samuels, C. (2023c, November 21). *How much does In-Home dementia care cost? Surprising facts and resources*. A Place For Mom .https://www.aplaceformom.com/caregiver-resources/articles/cost-of-dementia-care

Sauer, A. (2018, August 7). *Why do seniors want to stay in their homes?* Senior Living at Its Best | Leisure Care. https://www.leisurecare.com/resources/why-do-seniors-want-to-stay-home/

Sauer, A. (2023, April 19). *7 Technological innovations for those with dementia*. OurParents. https://www.ourparents.com/products-for-seniors/technology-for-dementia

7. *Ethical issues with residents with dementia.* (n.d.). A Train Education. https://www.atrainceu.com/content/7-ethical-issues-residents-dementia

Shu, S., & Woo, B. K. (2021). Use of technology and social media in dementia care: Current and future directions. *World Journal of Psychiatry, 11*(4), 109–123. https://doi.org/10.5498/wjp.v11.i4.109

Skilled Nursing Facility (SNF) care past 100 days. (2023, October 18). Medicare Interactive. https://www.medicareinteractive.org/get-answers/medicare-covered-services/skilled-nursing-facility-snf-services/snf-care-past-100-days

Sörensen, S., & Conwell, Y. (2011). Issues in Dementia Caregiving: effects on mental and physical health, intervention strategies, and research needs. *American Journal of Geriatric Psychiatry, 19*(6), 491–496. https://doi.org/10.1097/jgp.0b013e31821c0e6e

Stoddard Financial, LLC. (2023, May 2). *Planning for the costs of Alzheimer's and dementia care.* Stoddard Financial. https://www.stoddardfinancial.net/planning-dementia-alzheimers-care-cost/

Sturge, J., Klaassens, M., Jones, C., Elf, M., Weitkamp, G., & Meijering, L. (2021). *Exploring assets of people with memory problems and dementia in public space: A qualitative study.* Wellbeing, Space and Society, 2, 100063. https://doi.org/10.1016/j.wss.2021.100063

Success Stories. (n.d.). Homebridge | Quality In-home Care. https://www.homebridgeca.org/success-stories

Sullivan, S., & Sullivan, S. (2023, July 26). *How to apply for Medicare online – step by step.* USA Medicare Plan. https://usamedicareplan.com/how-to-apply-for-medicare-online/

Summers, L.E. (2023) *Compassionate Care: Navigating Dementia Together: How to be Confident and Informed in the Care of Your Loved One, Access Tools to Provide the Best Quality of Life, Maintain Your Work-Life Balance.* Goodreads. https://www.goodreads.com/book/show/199504859-compassionate-care

Support for people with dementia, including Alzheimer's disease. (n.d.). Administration for Community Living. http://acl.gov/programs/support-people-alzheimers-disease/support-people-dementia-including-alzheimers-disease

Technology and gadgets that make life easier for dementia patients and their caregivers. (n.d.). Visiting Angels. https://www.visitingangels.com/barrington/articles/technology-and-gadgets-that-make-life-easier-for-dementia-patients-and-their-caregivers/14417

Telehealth: Improving dementia care. (2020, September 23). National Institute on Aging. https://www.nia.nih.gov/news/telehealth-improving-dementia-care

Tips for managing caregiver stress. (2021, July 30). Alzheimer's Foundation of America. https://alzfdn.org/tips-for-managing-caregiver-stress/

30 meaningful moments – ideas for creating joy with those living with dementia. (2021, September 28). Life Circles.https://lifecircles-pace.org/30-meaningful-moments-ideas-for-creating-joy-with-those-living-with-dementia/

Tips for dementia-friendly documents. (n.d.). Alzheimer's Society. https://www.alzheimers.org.uk/dementia-professionals/dementia-experience-toolkit/real-life-examples/tips-dementia-friendly-documents

Topfer, L. (2016, August 31). *GPS locator devices for people with dementia.* CADTH Issues in Emerging Health Technologies - NCBI Bookshelf. https://www.ncbi.nlm.nih.gov/books/NBK391026/

Treatments and research. (n.d.). Alzheimer's Disease and Dementia. https://www.alz.org/help-support/i-have-alz/treatments-research

12 best GPS trackers for dementia patients | Family1st. (2023, December 6). Family1st. https://family1st.io/10-best-gps-trackers-for-dementia-patients/

25 Quick journal prompts that reduce caregiver stress and improve health. (2023b, December 19) DailyCaring. https://dailycaring.com/25-quick-journal-prompts-that-reduce-caregiver-stress-and-improve-health/

2024 Medicare parts A & B premiums and deductibles. (2023, October 12). Centers for Medicare & Medicaid Services. https://www.cms.gov/newsroom/fact-sheets/2024-medicare-parts-b-premiums-and-deductibles

Vail, C. (2021, December 30). *Engaging and fun video calls with family far away [15+ tips].* Grannies Go Digital. https://www.granniesgodigital.com/video-calls/tips-for-engaging-family-video-calls/

Van Dyk, D., & Dono, L. (2023, November 8). *Care tips to keep dementia patients safe at home.* AARP. https://www.aarp.org/caregiving/home-care/info-2017/dementia-home-safety.html

When is guardianship appropriate? (2022, August 18). Parentgiving. https://www.parentgiving.com/blogs/caregiving/when-is-guardianship-appropriate

Why future proofing dementia care requires partnerships to be built across the social care sector. (2022, May 23). Caring Times. https://caring-times.co.uk/feature/why-future-proofing-dementia-care-requires-partnerships-to-be-built-across-the-social-care-sector/

Wiese, J., Perrin, P. B., Aggarwal, R., Peralta, S. V., Stolfi, M. E., Morelli, E., Obeso, L. a. P., Arango-Lasprilla, J. C., & Trapp, K. (2015). Personal strengths and health related quality of life in dementia caregivers from Latin America. *Behavioural Neurology, 2015,* 1–8. https://doi.org/10.1155/2015/507196

Wong, C. (2023, November 9). 7 financial resources on how to pay for memory care. *Experience Care.* https://experience.care/blog/7-resources-how-to-pay-for-memory-care

Zhai, S., Chu, F., Tan, M., Chi, N., Ward, T. M., & Yuwen, W. (2023, May 19). Digital health interventions to support family caregivers: An updated systematic review. *Digital Health.* https://doi.org/10.1177/20552076231171967

125

Made in the USA
Coppell, TX
30 November 2024

41403634R00079